DOWN IN THE MOUTH AGAIN

A Dental Patient's Guide to
Everything They Should Know,
But Have No Idea.

DR. DEBORAH L. MARYNAK

DOWN IN THE MOUTH AGAIN

Cover and Interior Design by
Transcendent Publishing

TRANSCENDENT
publishing

ISBN: 979-8-218-06898-1

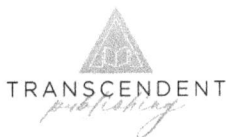

The author has made every effort to relay the stories in this book to be true and correct. They are written from the personal experiences of the author, friends, and colleagues. Both the author and the publisher disclaim any liability to any party for any loss or damage caused by errors or omissions.

Printed in the United States of America.

DEDICATION

This book is dedicated to a small group of people in the world who have dedicated their lives to the practice of treating dental disease. They wear many hats, and their role is quite impossible; they are managers, accountants, and marketers; they are business owners, plumbers, electricians, mechanics, *and* physicians of the mouth.

"Blessed are those who engage in lively debate with the helplessly mute, for they shall be called dentists."

—Ann Landers

CONTENTS

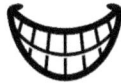

INTRODUCTION

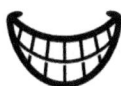

In my fifty-plus years in dentistry, I feel as if I've just about seen and heard it all. I cannot tell you how many times a dental professional has come up to me with another outrageous story from a patient who thinks we believe them. I know, I know it was your perception, but (probably) wrongly interpreted.

My years of experience and the like of my colleagues has ignited a passion. (You know it's a passion when you can't stop thinking about it.) This is the burning (and I mean *burning*) desire to educate the people – to raise their awareness of the importance of good dental health – to turn up the respect for these hardworking professionals (and their teams). To destroy the myths and put the absolute truth out there for the people to see. (Sorry, you're just going to have to suck it up and listen unless, of course, you want to keep blaming your dental issues on something other than yourself.)

This book aims to set the story straight...very straight. I hope it will be read by many dental professionals and that they are entertained. After all, it's dedicated to them! I'm certain they will find the humor – and, undoubtedly, similarities to stories of their own – and say to themselves, "Finally, someone is saying this out loud!"

My bigger dream, however, is to have this book read by the layperson, so they can understand the simple and obtainable objective of dental health. As the highly revered Dr. Eva Dahl once said to me, "A toothbrush and dental floss hold absolutely no socioeconomic barriers." Wow – now that's profound. Did you hear what she said? Dental health does not depend on how much money you do or do not have…all that matters is your attitude towards it.

I hope you will take from this book a much greater appreciation for the individual who sends you those reminder cards every three to six months. They work hard to get into dental school, harder to become dentists, and harder still to practice dentistry, so let's get on with it.

I have a lot to tell you.

CHAPTER ONE

DENTAL SCHOOL

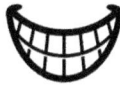

This is a good place to start. For some dental school was fun and for others it was torturous. When I went to school (from 1980 to 1984), it was absolute hell. Our triumphs and failures during pre-clinical practical testing (skills that were taught on fake teeth and fake patients) were laid out for all our classmates to see. Fortunately, I never endured the demeaning removal of the typodont head (the fake head with teeth in it) indicating you had, in fact, flunked the practical. (Bear with me here, this is for the dentists.)

I did, however, have the pain of watching my benchmates, people I had grown to love, endure the embarrassment of everyone in the class knowing they had not passed and would suffer the consequences. Ducking into the restroom to pray just before the practical became a ritual for me and many of my friends.

Fortunately, today's more stringent privacy laws put an end to this shameful practice of displaying failure for all to see. That said, there are still countless dentists around to tell the grueling tale, and even more patients who slide into their chairs with no idea what they went through for the privilege of working in this profession.

So here it is. Just like prospective medical school students, those planning on dental school must complete the required prerequisite classes, called "pre-dent," in math, physics, inorganic chemistry, organic chemistry, zoology, and animal biology, as well as English, art, psychology, and sociology. This is all before they can even think about applying to dental school. Then there's the Dental Admissions Test – now that was fun!

The Dental Admissions Test has four sections:

- Survey of Natural Sciences
- Reading Comprehension
- Quantitative Reasoning
- Perceptual Ability

These are reasonable tests to grant a wannabe dentist entrance to dental school, but the Perceptual Ability gave me a headache for two days! It examines your ability to visualize and manipulate objects mentally in three dimensions, as well as your skill in discriminating between angles that are very close in size. For someone to be able to determine changes in spatial relations, extremely minor differences in angles, or mentally manipulate objects, no problem! Suffice it to say, if you fail this section, forget it, you will not be going to dental school.

There was a small percentage of people who were accepted without a BS or a BA degree; however, these people weren't exempt from the pre-dent requirements. They had accumulated accomplishments well beyond the usual and customary dental school hopeful, such as practicing as dental assistants or dental hygienists, spending years working in a dental laboratory, or – in my case – all three.

I had classmates who were gifted clinically but not as book smart. Others didn't do well in the numerous laboratory classes but could ace any test on any subject. I was particularly good clinically, but I worked hard at most academics. Some classes were easier than others. If it was a visual thing, like dental anatomy, gross anatomy, or head and neck anatomy, I did very well. Other topics didn't come as easily, especially if they involved statistics or any sort of abstract information. Personally, I don't care about the dissociation of two chemicals in a beaker. If I can't see it, so what!

Even when it did come easily, I never walked around bragging about it or said about a test, "I didn't even have to study for it." I also never knew how to take these individuals who did brag because, truly, very little of dental school was easy, just as few things about operating a dental practice today are easy. Patients: please stop thinking of us as tooth technicians – it's disrespectful!

I recently had an electrician in my home who insisted dentists were being trained at his military base. I tried to explain that they are licensed Doctors of Dentistry doing a residency or simply working at a military facility. He seemed surprised. I had to tell him to achieve a license to practice dentistry in the U.S., one has to be trained, tested, and qualified by an accredited university, School of Dentistry.

I always said I was going to wallpaper a wall in my private office in tuition fee statements. Then, every time a patient complains about the cost of a crown, I'd take them into my office, sit them down and show them what it cost me to learn how to properly repair their teeth, diagnose a lesion, or treat their bone loss. Then I'd show them the drawings and the beautiful wax teeth I spent hundreds of hours drawing and carving only after I learned the name of every surface, cusp, groove, pit, indentation, and root of every adult and "baby" tooth, fifty-two teeth in all.

Did you know there were tests where we walked into the lab, were given a block of wax and a tooth number, and told to carve it perfectly from memory? How many people do you know who can do that? Let's be clear here: this is just dental anatomy…one class. I was one of the lucky ones – this just happened to be one of the classes I was good at. (There were many in which I struggled.) For those poor souls who weren't good at dental anatomy, and had to work *extremely hard*, it was grueling.

Dental anatomy was also one of the very first courses; if you didn't do well there, you were out, gone, asked to leave. You might say – and forgive my outdated lingo here – that it separated the men from the boys. The first couple of quarters weeded out anyone who didn't come in with an appropriate attitude – or aptitude. One of my bench mates was eliminated, went on to law school, and now represents – you got it – dentists.

Preclinical was that area where we practiced on fake mouths. (Some of us fondly recall this as "bench top dentistry.") This is where we learned how to do procedures while looking in a mirror. In fact, most of what we do is done while looking in a mirror – didn't know that did you? Pre-clinical was technically eighteen months, but you had to reach a certain level of proficiency before moving on to live patients. I remember students who started dental school one and two years before I did, only to linger in pre-clinical after I had moved on to live patients in clinical dentistry. Wow. Painful.

I recall a dental assistant who worked in my private practice asking me what lab I had used as a student to construct my patients' restorations. (Those gold crowns, inlays and onlays we prepped, impressioned, then constructed ourselves, and placed into our patients' mouths.) I laughed and told her that, except for porcelain crowns, I did my own lab work. (In dental school we had to do so many surfaces of silver fillings, gold restorations, porcelain crowns, dentures, partials, etc.) Then she asked where we got our dental assistants from, and I laughed again. There were assistants in every clinic, but they only occasionally stepped in to help with mixing impression material; otherwise, we did everything ourselves.

Anyway, I guess even those days are over. When I went to dental school, to take an impression, we expressed two parts of material and mixed it on a mixing pad, then loaded a syringe to take an impression. Today there are impression materials that are preloaded in a special "gun-like apparatus" with mixing tips. The gun expresses two materials and as they enter the mixing tip the two materials are scientifically mixed, doing all the work for us. Easy-peasy!

This may not mean anything to you, but working without an assistant is extremely hard. You try working backward in a mirror with the patient's hot breath fogging it up and water spraying everywhere. Go ahead…try it. Then add the patient moving, looking at his cell phone (How rude!), bringing his hands up (How stupid…our instruments are sharp!), jiggling his feet (Hello…when you jiggle your feet, your head moves.) Sit still!

The science portion of the Dental Boards came toward the end of the second of our four years. I recall the room well. We sat in this extremely large room with one hundred and forty, six-foot-long tables with one chair at each table. I guess they assumed we were going to cheat, and this was a way to insure we could not see our neighbor's answer sheet. If I remember correctly, it was two eight-hour days of testing in histology, microbiology, human anatomy and physiology, embryology, biochemistry, and the like. Oh, and I know what you're thinking…

You're wondering why a dentist would have to know these topics if they just work on teeth. I just can't wrap my head around these types of questions as they seem so profoundly stupid to me. It's as if the teeth are a separate entity from the remainder of the body. Teeth are just these white, hard structures that get cavities and occasionally need repair. So, let's have a little science lesson.

If we must know all about teeth, it's important for us to know where they come from, or how we get them. In studying embryology, we learn that *all* tissues and structures in the body come from three "germ layers": endoderm, mesoderm, and ectoderm. This is where teeth come from as well and all three germ layers are responsible for the formation of the teeth, bone, ligament, muscles, nerves, and blood supply. Since there are developmental anomalies during fetal development that affect teeth, I guess it may be important to study embryology.

Histology is important because it is the study of the various tissues that make up the body. Teeth have several kinds of tissue. There's the outer portion of the tooth that is hard tissue and the inner portion (pulp chamber) that is soft tissue. Both parts of the tooth come from various germ layers and when nature goes wrong with certain germ layers, it may affect the teeth.

Most people know that teeth can get infected, and since we need to know how to treat infections, I'm thinking an understanding of biochemistry and physiology is in order. For those two sciences to make any sense, we'd have to understand human anatomy. (We spent six months dissecting the human body.)

I remember an instructor telling me, "If you think dental school is hard, just wait until you get out." At the time, I thought he was just being funny; never did I imagine what was ahead for me.

CHAPTER TWO

I GRADUATED, NOW WHAT?

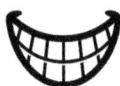

O nce you graduate, you take the second set of boards – the clinical board. This is where you get to do some dentistry and it's judged for competency. You find your own patients, and if they are from out of town you pay for their travel, food, and housing. This was especially upsetting to the forty percent of my class who failed the periodontology portion of the board. Those students had to travel from Minnesota to Kansas to retake it – again, all on their own dime. Talk about stressful!

I'm not certain how that all turned out for them, I was just grateful I didn't have to do it. I recall standing at my mailbox with my board results in my hand, petrified to open it and incredibly grateful once I did and learned I'd passed. Then there was the jurisprudence exam testing your knowledge of the laws, rules, and regulations that govern your State Board of Dentistry. Pay for your license, obtain some malpractice insurance and *now* you're eligible to start practicing dentistry – but where?

We had all given thought to the several choices we had as licensed professionals; however, while some already had jobs, others wanted to stop and ponder their opportunities. I could specialize, but that would mean another two to four years of education…and more debt – no thanks. Next question: should I work for someone else, or start my own practice?

The problem with going out on my own was the cost which, added to student loans, would result in a staggering amount of debt. In today's world, it's close to a million dollars; I only know this because I have a couple of friends fresh out of dental school. One of them purchased an existing practice and the other started his own practice. Heaven forbid they married someone from their class with their own student loan debt – it would take forever to get out from under that burden.

And that's just the financial aspect. As I would soon learn, dental school deserved a big fat F when it came to preparing me and my classmates to practice dentistry. Most of us graduated with no knowledge or skills necessary to either run or be part of a successful business. Furthermore, success depends on the creation of an outstanding office culture. It is imperative to create a culture where dental teams enjoy coming to work and they, in turn, help create happy, paying patients who return year after year. Patients feel everything (good and bad) going on in our dental practices, and if you are unable to create that happy culture, you can expect to fail at some point.

That said, outstanding office culture, as important as it is, is only a fraction of what's necessary to succeed in dentistry. Problems will come in all shapes and sizes, so like my instructor said: "if you think this is hard, wait until you get out."

I recall the patient who was shocked when we asked for her co-pay. She looked at her young daughter and said, "I guess we're not getting a Christmas tree this year because Dr. Marynak needs to be paid." I came out of my office and asked if there was a problem. When I explained I had policies she'd agreed to as we were running a business, she gasped and stated that dentistry wasn't a "business," it was a "healthcare responsibility."

How would you handle this? At that time, I didn't know what to say. I knew what I wanted to say, but it would have been inappropriate! Decades later I can say this:

Patients: Every aspect of healthcare is a business; dentistry is no exception.

Dentists: If you are unable to run your practice as a business, you'll never flourish. Your work will simply become an albatross.

Chapter Three

YOU'RE NOT A REAL DOCTOR

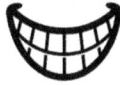

O ne day after work I headed to the underground garage to retrieve my car. When I said to the attendant, "Dr. Marynak, please," he asked, "What kind of a doctor are you?" I told him that I was a Doctor of Dentistry," and was met with a smirk. "Oh," he said, "you're not a *real* doctor." I just smiled, got into my car, and went home.

About two months later, I was in the garage, rummaging through my purse as I waited for the attendant. "Dr. Marynak, please," I said, and looked up to see the same young man, now with a very swollen cheek and an eye that was starting to swell shut as well. He stated he was thinking he should find me as he was getting a toothache. I recommended he see a "real doctor."

This story is not unique; in fact, in one form or another it's probably as old as the practice of dentistry itself, with comments like, "You're not a *real* doctor" or "You're *just* a dentist" rolling easily off the tongue. So why is it that when the author of this book went to the ER in small-town Wisconsin for a toothache.

(Prior to my dental education I did not understand or heed the importance of home care and now it had caught up to me.) the MD had *absolutely no idea* how to treat said toothache?

After I told her the tooth number (Damn, they don't even know tooth numbers?), the diagnosis, the pain meds, and the name and dose of the proper antibiotic, the MD billed me – are you ready? – *three hundred and eighty-seven dollars*! To make matters worse, she poked her head into the exam room and asked if this dentist with tooth pain "was a joke?" Hello! I wasn't born a dentist and the last time I cut my finger, it bled!

The next time you hear someone spout off that dentists aren't *real* doctors, tell them the next time they get a toothache to go to their medical doctor and see if they can get help there. They won't, because MDs know zero about dental disease...zero. I speak from experience on this, having never seen a patient successfully treated by an MD for a toothache. If, like me, they head to an emergency room because it's after-hours, they wind up in my office, still swollen and in pain, three days later. What's more, in a hundred percent of these cases (and there have been dozens of them), they've also been given the wrong prescription.

I tell you this because I worked in a welfare clinic in an area where there is no water fluoridation. [1]Drugs and free healthcare

---

[1] By the time we reach adulthood, a good share of our dental damage has been done, especially if we didn't have the good fortune of being raised in a fluoridated community. Oh no! I said the "f" word...fluoride! News flash...any substance can be considered a poison if it's taken improperly!! Water can kill you if you drink too much of it. You *will* benefit from about .7 parts fluoride per million parts water as your teeth develop. And you will benefit from those fluoride treatments your hygienist wants to give you. Now get over it. Really. Truth be known, you just don't want to pay for it.

bring a multitude of dental and medical problems. Patients were regularly seen a day or two after receiving meds in the emergency room from medical doctors because they were still in pain.

It positively torques my chain when someone asks why a dental student needs to dissect the human body during their training. Or how about the elderly couple who left my practice because I gave them an oral cancer exam, stating, "I was working outside of my area of expertise." Ignorance!

It's not just everyday people who say these things, but our medical colleagues as well. In fact, the first time I heard it, the individual was a pre-med student with whom I was attending pre-dent classes. He teased and laughed as he explained that all we do is "tinker with teeth" – no matter his own father was a dentist!

I started distancing myself from him because of his disrespectful view of what it means to become a physician of the mouth, head, and neck. I do recall him saying that they only spent four hours studying the mouth. That was in the early eighties. My niece, a pathologist in a large hospital in Omaha, said they spent zero hours studying the mouth in medical school. That was in the first decade of 2000.

I've no idea where this medical doctor is today, but I can assume he isn't a famous clinician revered for heroic deeds. There are no medical magazines with his face adorning the cover, no written articles about how he has changed the world or is saving lives. Yet I'll wager he still holds the same superior attitude when it comes to dentists as he did back in premed.

Then there was the CEO of a large corporate medical facility to whom I reached out about an issue I'd experienced in one of the clinics. Upon returning my call, he'd asked what kind of doctor I was, as I'd referred to myself in my message as "Dr. Marynak." When I told him I was a doctor of dentistry, he became very rude, dismissive, and arrogant. His comment was, "Oh, you're a *den*-tist." – as if it held no significance whatsoever.

Recently, a friend of mine had some dental work done in Mexico. Now I cautioned her about doing this, but she assured me that this dentist had trained in the United States. My friend also has a background in dentistry, having worked in dental offices, off and on, her entire adult life, so I knew she wasn't going into this blind.

During one of her visits, this dentist revealed why he preferred practicing in Mexico. He told her that in Mexico, dentists are revered and highly respected, as opposed to the United States, where they are treated like second-class citizens compared to medical doctors. "Dentists in the U.S.," he said, "are considered milk toast."

Interesting.

In all professions, there are the good, the great, and the "oh, my!" That said, there are physicians who practice basic medicine – wellness exams, ordering tests, reading the results, and prescribing medications – and know when to refer the patient out for a higher level of care. My opinion, of course, but there is no real difficulty in doing these things – it's simply a matter of training.

A well-trained general dentist, on the other hand, knows how to prepare your crooked teeth for crowns and make them turn out to be perfectly straight. These procedures can change a patient's smile and, ultimately, their life. How about the guys who can place an implant after they've done the surgery to lift the maxillary sinus cavity and increase the girth of bone so it can support that implant?

Milk toast…? I think not.

I know I've never felt like milk toast when I finished a large cosmetic case and handed my patient a mirror to see them burst out in tears of joy. And I've certainly never felt that way when they jump up, hug me, and say, "I never thought I could look like this. Thank you!"

Of course, with that ability comes a tremendous amount of pressure and responsibility. In fact, that's the primary reason dental hygienists give me (and I've asked many) for not going on to dental school as I did. I also had a friend who told me his one goal was to become an outstanding cosmetic dentist. Over dinner one evening, I recommended a course I had taken, and he immediately enrolled. Unfortunately, partway through the clinical portion of the course, the instructor told him he didn't have what it took to become a cosmetic dentist. One day shortly after that, my friend put a gun in his mouth and pulled the trigger. Getting the picture?

All this is to say, "When is America going to view us differently?" I know, I know, some people *do* see us as real physicians of the mouth, but we're a long way from equal respect. Moreover, many patients don't understand or think about everything we handle, starting with pre-dent, dental school, dental practice, continual training, and debt, debt, debt. Personally, I think we should all go to medical school and dentistry should simply be a specialty of medicine. This won't be the last time I say this, and it won't happen in my lifetime!

Dentists have sacrificed a lot for the privilege of providing you with good dental treatment, so, to conclude this rant, I'll ask you to be the best dental patient you can for them – for example:

1. Stop canceling your appointments, showing up late, or, worse yet, just failing to show up at all. (In fact, come early so you can use the bathroom beforehand!)

2. If you do show up late, don't expect to complete the planned treatment. No one on the schedule should have to wait because of your failure to plan.

3. Stop choosing to do the procedure that's less expensive and, when it fails, expecting us to redo it at no charge because your insurance only pays for it every two years.

4. Expect to pay your bill at the door.

5. Turn off your phone, sit still, and open your mouth. To do anything else makes our already difficult job that much harder.

CHAPTER FOUR

THE PURPOSE AND IMPORTANCE OF YOUR TEETH

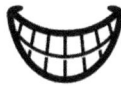

I often wonder where the disconnect between our teeth and our overall health comes from. I can't tell you how many people, upon learning the cost of a root canal treatment, say, "Just take it out!" Then it's my job to inform them of the cascading problems they may face in the future if they elected in the moment to save money and get an extraction.

Of those who don't listen, many say they'll get an implant "at some point." Rarely do I see follow-through; however, I do see all the things that I explained would happen start to happen. One of these things is the teeth start to "tip and drift." You see, the teeth hold each other in place – and not only the teeth next to each other; the upper teeth hold the lowers down and vice versa. If you lose a tooth and the adjacent teeth start to tip into the now vacant space, the opposing teeth will start to drift into the space the opposing tooth left by tipping. Not to mention the problem chewing if you keep losing teeth!

Patients tell me they get by "just fine," and that's when I know they don't really understand the importance and purpose of their teeth. They're not there just so you can smile, folks! Lose those back teeth and that smile will slowly start to fall apart. How, you ask?

Without molars, the remaining teeth have to do more work to chew food. Since digestion of fats and carbohydrates begins in the mouth, emulsification of food is incredibly important. Food that is not fully readied for the stomach can't nourish your body as well as it could if those molars were there to do the work for which they were designed.

I've seen hundreds of patients go down the path of losing their back teeth and expecting their front teeth to chew their food. News flash: God did not design the teeth in the front of your mouth to chew your food. These teeth cannot sustain the work designed for the molars. They were designed to cut and tear, not chew! How long do you think they can sustain that type of abuse and survive?

Years of improperly chewing your food, coupled with poor eating habits, will affect your longevity. As you lose teeth, the food you choose will be softer and easier to chew, leading to any number of medical issues. I'll say it again: early loss of your teeth has been shown to lead to increased medical problems and earlier death. The worst part (but the good news) is that it's all preventable.

How about the topic of speech? Sit in a quiet room and talk out loud to yourself. Notice the movement of your tongue against your teeth as you work to form your words. Maybe you are doing this exercise and some of your words are more difficult to form because you're missing some of your dentition. Are you getting the picture yet?

Your teeth are an amazing tool designed for beauty, communication, and health. Start losing them and you'll also eventually start to lose your beautiful smile, your ability to communicate clearly, and your health!

CHAPTER FIVE

THE BUSINESS OF
PRACTICING DENTISTRY

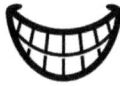

T here are many types of dental practices (I've worked in almost all of them, in case you're wondering where my opinions come from), including corporate practices, Indian Healthcare, private solo practices, group practices, nursing home practices, mobile practices, prison dentistry, and Veterans' Affairs (VA) dentistry – just to name a few. Some states allow denture practices that are owned by a denturist and employ a dentist for any needed dental work (i.e., extractions, fillings, cleanings, and/or crowns) prior to placement of partials and dentures. The more providers there are, the greater the number of support staff you need; the more staff you have, the more problems you have as well.

I recall being surprised when a colleague/friend said to me, "I don't care who you are or what you do, there is no occupation that is more difficult than the practice of dentistry." Upon reflection, however, I realize I totally agree with that statement. No matter what venue you work in, clinical dentistry is extremely hard work; that said, there is nothing more difficult than owning your own practice.

Another colleague/friend had a dad and an uncle who were dentists. He told me he used to get mad at his father for coming from a long day at his practice and falling asleep on the couch instead of engaging with him. It wasn't until years later, when he had his own dental practice, that he understood how exhausting it was.

Let's look at a list of issues that every dental practice owner must deal with, then we'll get into the expenses specific to a practice owner.

1. Hiring
2. Firing
3. Staff reviews
4. Staff raises
5. Staff discipline
6. Creating/updating an office manual on practice expectations, rules, and regulations
7. HIIPA/Harassment Prevention/Medicare Fraud/Cultural Competency review
8. Procedural documentation
9. Insurance documentation
10. New patient photography
11. Medical releases
12. Chart review

This list doesn't look long (and I'm certain I've left out something), but it amounts to a mountain of issues that need continuous attention. Add these all together PLUS producing dentistry...ugh! This is the reason dentists go into corporate dentistry, Indian Healthcare, community service, VA dentistry, etc., etc. When you don't own the business and work as an employee, the problems are different... and far fewer. Enter the Dental Office Manager!

A well-tuned practice utilizes an office manager who can deal with these long lists, freeing up the dentist to do his/her most important job: producing dentistry. I'm always concerned when I enter a dental practice, ask for the manager, and hear, "We don't really have an office manager." I get a headache just thinking about how tired the practice owner must be and/ or the myriad fires that are being left unattended.

And then there are the expenses...

Most patients think we charge too much, but I know of none who has even an inkling of the cost of doing dentistry. Below are some of them; again; I'm certain I've missed a few, but this should give you an idea of what it takes to hang out that shingle.

1. Rent or mortgage payment on the building
2. Real estate taxes (if you own the building)
3. Utilities
4. Malpractice insurance
5. Doctor's continuing education
6. Team's continuing education

7. Team uniforms

8. Payroll

9. Payroll taxes

10. Workers' Compensation Insurance

11. Clinical supplies

12. Office supplies

13. Dental software program/support

14. Professional association dues

15. Telephone and answering services

16. Leased equipment

17. Student loans

18. Dental license

19. Narcotics license (DEA)

20. Marketing

21. Employee benefits

22. Dental lab bills

23. Quarterly taxes

24. Website/website support

Yes, it's a business, though few of us hold a business degree or received any training on how to run it. My point is this: think about all this the next time you want to balk at paying a portion of your dental bill.

I recall, in the not-too-distant past, a patient telling me the cost of a crown was "ridiculous." Today, most crowns cost somewhere in the range of $900 to $1200, and even up to $2500 or more depending on where you receive treatment. They should last about eight to twenty years, depending on how well they are done and how well they are cared for by their owners. When was the last time you spent that kind of money on your car and had it last that long? If I put it to you like that, does it still sound ridiculous?

If the man in Chapter Three took a moment to think about it, I'm pretty sure he would not have made such an ignorant (and insulting) statement. He couldn't have considered the overhead involved in running a practice, and certainly not the time and money dentists spend on their training, as well as continuing education and licensure fees. As you can see above, the list of expenses is endless – and, for most individuals, would be a shock to the system.

As I've stated before, *most* dentists are notoriously poor businesspeople; that said, the ones who are good at business do extremely well. In today's world, it's customary practice to have the patient pay their portion of the cost at the end of their appointment. However, when I diagnosed a cosmetic treatment plan costing $10,000 to $50,000, I required half down just to make the first appointment. The second half was due before we sat you in the chair to begin treatment. As soon as I incurred cost, you were going to incur cost, and that pretty much assured me you were going to show up.

In most states, you must have treatment plans signed by the patient prior to treatment. If treatment is started without that signature, patients don't have to pay anything. It also means that if you start an irreversible procedure on a patient you are bound to finish that procedure, irrespective of whether or not they intend to pay for the treatment. Today: no signed treatment plan, then no treatment and no prepayment – no appointment, period!

Incredibly, I have gone into dental offices to find they are still not obtaining a signed treatment plan! A signature doesn't bind the patient to get the work completed. It's simply a form of risk management stating the patient has been fully informed regarding the recommended treatment, risks, and alternatives. The patient's questions have been asked and answered, and they are fully informed of the cost involved and how it was to be paid.

Again, depending on the state where you practice dentistry, signed treatment plans are a basic requirement prior to beginning any treatment. When I was in private practice in Minnesota, the rules went like this: without, a signed treatment plan, the patient could look you in the eye and refuse to pay for the treatment; the clinician was bound to complete anything that had been started and was irreversible, with or without payment. Lessons learned!

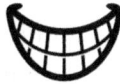

CHAPTER SIX

DENTAL AUXILIARIES

Dental assistants, dental hygienists, receptionists, and office managers – this is the small army of people who make the office function and without whom no dentistry is done. There are the good ones, the outstanding ones, the bad, and the ugly. I've met them all! As in most fields, there are only a handful of outstanding ones; they are there to do a stellar job and have no time for gossipers, lazy colleagues, or any sort of nonsense. They are best described like this:

They show up to work a little early to be sure they were prepared for the huddle. During the huddle they're attentive to any prospective problems to the schedule and they bring solutions to the problems. They possess a sense of urgency in their work, as is often needed in the practice of Dentistry.

They're able to think outside the box and easily prioritized issues as they arise. They can thoroughly turn a room at a moment's notice and pick up slack whenever needed. They've memorized the doctor's procedures and systems; they're considered his or her "right arm." In short, they can be counted on to be there and when they're not in the office, their absence can be felt by the entire team.

In the company of patients, they always have a smile on their face. They listen and document everything exactly as described to them. They don't share personal issues with patients, but they listen when patients share their personal problems.

They remember the patient's names, families' names, and personal interests. They are fully engaged!

Then there are the employees who show up late to the huddle with their hair still wet and their scrubs all wrinkled. They can't seem to function without their phone within arm's length. They're the first to lunch and the first to leave at the end of the day. They are the ones who make more work for the rest of the team. They are wonderful with patients and kind to their colleagues, which is the only thing saving their jobs. As the saying goes, you're only as strong as your weakest link, and employees like this will weaken the whole practice.

Now, for all you practice owners out there, let's try to find the right people to create the support team. Not an easy task since you were never trained to hire employees. Personally, I wasn't good at it and struggled when I owned my private practice. Today, there are many tools and individuals who can help place the right people in your path, but again, those people – you got it – cost money. Are you starting to see why crowns cost so much? And we've barely scratched the surface!

I'd like to take this time to give a shoutout to the handful of great women (and some men) for the privilege of having worked with them. If they are reading this, they know who they are because I've told them, and I remain their friend and biggest fan. They are the ones who were on my mind when I wrote what makes up what I consider a rock star dental auxiliary. Thank you, my dental favorites. I think of you often and I'm so grateful you crossed my path!

Chapter Seven

THE RELATIONSHIP BETWEEN MEDICINE AND DENTISTRY

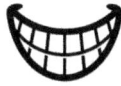

Patients are often surprised when we ask them about their current medical conditions and medications, and even more so when we tell them to include herbal supplements.

As I've shared, in dental school we dissected the human body, studied physiology, biochemistry, microbiology, embryology, and histology, to name a few. The common response to that is, "Why do you need to study all of that when you're just going to work on my teeth?" Last time I checked; your teeth are attached to the systems that operate your entire body. Therefore, as dental professionals, we must know and understand the medications and medical conditions of all patients we treat.

Here are a couple of examples:

- If you're diabetic, we should know your A1C. If your A1C isn't seven or less, we will struggle to control your periodontal disease.

- If you've taken any anticoagulants and need a tooth removed, we need to know. We'll need to consult with your MD, so when we ask for their name and phone number, we mean it.
- If you need an infected tooth removed, we need to know if you have any allergies; antibiotics prior to an extraction help the anesthetic work better.
- If you are being treated for osteoporosis and are taking any bisphosphonates, removing a tooth can cause the failure of the bone to heal.
- If you have a damaged, repaired, or replaced heart valve, you need antibiotics prior to your dental appointment.

Again, teeth are not a separate entity from the rest of your body. So often, patients think they know more than we do; I would encourage any dentist to dismiss those types of patients – they're a liability.

In the fifty-plus years I have been in the field of dentistry, I have seen a direct correlation between the premature loss of teeth and the decline of health; premature loss of teeth, and early death. You do it to yourself when you choose to take the tooth out instead of fixing it. I often hear, "It's in the back... no one will see it, no one will ever know!" Let me tell you this: your body knows.

Let's review it again: removing the tooth instead of treating and retaining it decreases your mouth's ability to properly chew food and get it digested to a point where your body can continue to digest it in your stomach and absorb the necessary nutrients your body needs. Thus, premature loss of teeth has a direct correlation to a decrease in optimal health, leading to an earlier-than-necessary death.

Physicians are causing problems about which they know nothing. They prescribe medications that are causing devastating oral conditions. I'm not saying these meds are unnecessary, however, MDs do little to prevent the dental disease they cause due to the condition known as "dry mouth." It's really scary how little medical doctors know about the mouth!

I had one MD tell me that it's like looking into a "deep, dark, mysterious hole." If that's not evidence of the ignorance regarding the connection between medical and dental health, I don't know what is.

Simply put, when saliva flow is decreased due to medications (and there are over four thousand of them that cause this), dental disease will rise – and cause horrific problems in patients with poor and marginal oral hygiene. Is it too much to ask that they understand the disease they're promoting and work with us to impress upon the patient's mind the absolute necessity of seeing a dentist more often than they normally would? At the very least, they could prescribe saliva substitutes to help prevent dental disease. Too often, we meet the patient after so much damage has been done and we're chasing our tail to reverse it.

Again, the mouth is where digestion of carbohydrates and fats begins. If you don't have your full dentition and appropriate saliva flow, properly chewing your food isn't possible, which impedes digestion and impairs the absorption of nutrients and weakens the entire body. Furthermore, a dry mouth increases the colonization of bacteria. When I see a patient with a filthy mouth, I wonder how much of the bacterial load in their mouth is taxing their immune system.

That said, some more fully informed MDs are getting up to speed, for example:

- Heart surgeons are now asking that patients get periodontal examinations and have specific periodontal bacteria reduced to a manageable number prior to open-heart surgery. Failure to do this can cause the surgery to fail over time.

- Diabetic patients who are struggling to control blood sugar are being examined for periodontal disease because we now know that periodontal bacteria and control of blood sugar are closely related.

- We have now found some of the nastier bacteria found in periodontal disease in the plaques that form in arteries and in the joints of patients with rheumatoid arthritis.

- I just finished a continuing education course on the genetic, autoimmune disorder Celiac Disease. This disorder can cause tooth deformities, teeth that don't harden properly, and an increased risk for dry mouth, both causing an increase in cavities, delayed tooth eruption and lower jaw deformities. [2]

Perhaps you now see why I believe dentistry isn't simply a specialty of medicine? That's the case in veterinary medicine, so

---

[2] Oral Manifestations of Celiac Disease; The Journal of Multidisciplinary Care; Decisions in Dentistry; March 2020Volume 6, Number 3; Jennifer S. Sherry, RDH, MSEd, Danna Cotner, DDS, Joel Hamilton, RD, LDN

why should it be different for those of us without four feet and fur? We don't just tinker with teeth, people. We're responsible for looking at the full picture.

I can't tell you how many times I'm reviewing medications and note the high number of patients with migraine prescriptions. On examining the patient and asking some questions, this is what I most often find:

1. Their masseter muscles are overly developed. These are one of the three muscles of closure. I can tell when a patient chews more on one side of their mouth because one side is more developed than the other.
2. I palpate the lateral pterygoid muscle and the patient winces…hmmm…telling. The second muscle of closure.
3. The teeth are flat and worn.
4. The patient reports the pain comes at the temples and up around the eyes.

This leads me to believe that these are not true migraines, but neuromuscular headaches caused by clenching and grinding either while sleeping or awake or both. I would suggest try- ing a thermoflex, flat-planed, canine-guided nightguard; I bet they'll sleep better, their headaches will subside, and they can stop taking meds. Do physicians ever think of this possibility? If so, it's a rarity.

I have a dear friend who was working in a state where patients on state aid are treated according to some rather strict rules. One of those rules went like this: if the dental practitioner found a suspicious oral lesion, it had to be referred to an MD, rather than an oral surgeon, for a diagnosis and determination as to whether it should be biopsied.

The following statistics are from the Oral Cancer Foundation:

"Close to 54,000 Americans will be diagnosed with oral or oropharyngeal cancer this year. It will cause over 9,750 deaths, killing roughly 1 person per hour, 24 hours per day. Of those 54,000 newly diagnosed individuals, only slightly more than half (approximately 57%) will be alive in 5 years. This is a number that has not significantly improved in decades." [3]

Comparing these facts to the rule in my friend's state, I can only conclude that state does not value their general dentists and oral surgeons as true physicians of the mouth. Having many friends in medicine, and knowing they study little or nothing regarding the oral cavity, I would not be comfortable sending my patients to an MD for a definitive diagnosis.

Years ago, I was having dinner with a former dental school classmate of mine, and we got on the topic of oral cancer exams. I told her I didn't have time to do oral cancer exams on my patients. She went on to tell me she'd missed a lesion on her mother that led to a radical neck dissection; although disfiguring, it was a life-saving procedure. Her only response to me was, "Make time." Her story compelled me to always, always, always, do the exam. If you're not getting an oral cancer exam at your dental check-ups, either ask for one or find a dentist who does them.

---

[3] Oral Cancer Facts. https://oralcancerfoundation.org/facts/#:~:text=Rates%20 of%20occurrence%20in%20the,be%20alive%20in%205%20years.

I had another friend, a heart surgeon, ask me: "Deb, are you aware that periodontal disease and heart disease were related?" My response was: "Don, we've known that for over ten years. We're just waiting for you guys to catch up!"

CHAPTER EIGHT

MY DENTIST IS AWESOME...

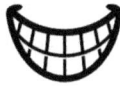

I've often wondered how people know their dentist is "awesome." Really, how do they know what kind of a dentist is treating them? Are they simply judging how well they get along? Would you be surprised to know that the level of skill with which they treat patients has everything to do with how they were raised or what *formed* their ethics and morals?

My belief is that most patients, especially male patients, choose their dentist based on their belief that they are comrades. When they visit their dentist, they laugh and share stories and behave as if they're friends. Perhaps they golf together, fish together, or hunt together; this builds friendship and trust, but unfortunately, it has nothing to do with skill or how well the dentist does his or her job. It does, however, create a stream of referrals.

Now I'm not inferring that happy, friendly dentists aren't good and even GREAT dentists, I'm simply stating a fact: a jovial personality may make the visit more pleasant, but it does not indicate the work performed is exceptional. On the flip side:

you can be a highly skilled clinician, but possess a crabby, angry, seemingly unhappy, or unfriendly personality, and patients and your staff will not want to be in the same room with you.

I have a friend who used to be a high school track and cross-country coach. I'd always enjoyed going to his meets, and on one occasion had the opportunity to meet his lead athlete, whose performance I had witnessed over the course of a year. My friend had spoken often about his abilities, as well as his desire to one day be a dentist. I too had observed his strength and speed; however, I also found him to be an incredibly angry young man.

His anger clouded his considerable athletic talent, and it became uncomfortable just to be around him as he always appeared "pissed." I told his coach that until he changed his demeanor, he needed to put dental school on the back burner. It's a tough enough way to make a living without one's personality making it harder.

Make no mistake about it: You can be the most clinically gifted Doctor of Dentistry that ever picked up a handpiece, but without some happiness in your personality, you **will** starve.

I feel it's important to stress that a dentist's personality has *absolutely nothing* to do with how skilled they are at performing dentistry. I've been told by many consultants (more on them later) that one can tell a dentist's skill level by the type of cars they drive, the type of office they work in, or the brand of watch they wear. I'm in complete disagreement with this. If you want to find a dentist who's a good businessperson, look at their watch and their car. If you want to find a highly skilled dentist, find a high-end dental laboratory or a popular special-ist of some kind and ask them to recommend a skilled dentist. They know when someone is the real deal.

Bottom line: if personality is important when it comes to how you feel about going to the dentist, that's your choice; just make sure it's not a substitute for their ability to place a crown, fill a cavity, diagnose a lesion, or treat periodontal disease.

CHAPTER NINE

THE GREAT, THE GOOD AND
THE NOT SO MUCH

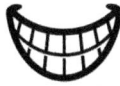

I've seen a lot of dentistry (By perhaps numerous of fellow clinicians), most of which is termed "clinically acceptable." Therefore, when I see work that is truly exceptional, I am compelled to ask the patient, "Who did this work...it's beautiful." It is so visually stimulating, it makes my brain sing. "Ugly" dentistry, on the other hand, makes my eyes hurt. It too makes me wonder who could have thought this passed for dentistry. *This crown doesn't fit! The margins are open, the color is horrific. Whoever this person is, they must have failed dental anatomy."*

As the name of this chapter suggests, I believe there are three levels of dentistry: the great, the good, and the not so much. If I knew any of my work fell in the not so much category, I'd redo it at no charge to the patient. I simply could not look at it at every six-month exam and feel good about myself. This, due in large part to the fact that I was raised by a woman who drove home the concept of giving one hundred and ten percent. That said, there are often extenuating circumstances, outside the control of the dentist, that play a role in how well a procedure is done.

Did the patient show up on time for the designated procedure? Is their oral hygiene good enough for us to control hemorrhage? Are they compliant? Compliance includes many issues. Do they moan during the procedure? Believe it or not, moaning affects us because we're human and, contrary to popular belief, we did not become dentists just to hurt people.

Do they keep moving their head and feet? Do they keep bringing their hands up to their face? Do they have long facial hair that I have to look through in order to work? Is their phone pinging and ringing? Did they bring a friend for emotional support who keeps interfering? These are just a few of the issues I've dealt with while trying to do my best, and obstacles to excellent care.

Of course, there are factors that involve the dentist. There were students in dental school who turned whatever they touched to gold and there were students whose work was simply acceptable; there were also those who were held back year after year due to clinical incompetence.

There was one student in my class who was a real genius. The way his brain worked and how he flew through tests without even blinking was amazing. The problem was he had zero manual dexterity. He must have had some visual acuity, or he wouldn't have passed the Dental Admissions Test; however, in dentistry you must be able to use your clinical knowledge, your visual acuity, and your manual dexterity together to complete treatment. And it needs to be done as quickly and efficiently as possible for the comfort of the patient.

In dentistry, like any endeavor, I believe that to go from good to great you must abandon any form of laziness and persevere, muster all your patience, and – perhaps most of all – possess a desire to get great! Newt Gingrich said, "Perseverance is the hard work you do after getting tired of doing the hard work you already did." To that, I say, "Amen!"

Chapter Ten

THE BOARD OF DENTISTRY, DOCUMENTATION, AND RISK MANAGEMENT

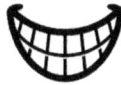

Ah, the Board of Dentistry... I have a strong opinion regarding this group of individuals who serve as the "police" of the dental profession. I don't always think they act appropriately. They often display an attitude of superiority and think they can say or do anything they please, that they are all-powerful. You know the type.

Now, hear me out: I understand that in the interest of public safety there must be policing of all professional individuals. Indeed, there's a board for everything from cosmetologists to pharmacists, nurses and dentists, medical doctors, chiropractors, and optometrists. I also know there are dental professionals who go astray, and I mean *way* astray. You'll see insurance fraud, drug use, poor risk management, practicing with an expired license, and on and on. But I don't believe that's the majority.

If I were a betting woman, I would guess that most of these are complaints from patients who don't want to pay their bill. A colleague of mine said, "People can always find fault with your work when they owe you money." Profound! If you want to hurt your provider, just complain to the Board of Dentistry. Just know that if your complaint is unfounded, it'll go nowhere. Most boards don't judge the quality of a practitioner's work either; that's for an ethics committee, peer review, or a malpractice attorney.

At one point I was working for a denture clinic that was under investigation by the Dental Board; they, along with the attorney general, were working to indict the woman who ran the clinic on behalf of her husband. I knew things weren't on the up and up, as she was constantly trying to dictate treatment. Problem was, she wasn't the doctor – I was. I didn't last long in her employment; no way was I going to jeopardize my license.

The Board sent two members to my new employer, asking for me. When they learned it was my day off, they asked where I lived and how far away it was; they needed to speak to me. My manager called me at home and told me what had happened, then gave me a number to call. As I picked up the phone, I couldn't imagine what I had done that necessitated their walking into my place of employment. They didn't answer, and they never called me back.

When I went to work the next day, everyone was looking at me sideways, as if I'd done something horribly wrong. When I finally did connect with the board members, they told me they had questions for me regarding the woman who ran the clinic where I was formerly employed. In response, I asked them point-blank if they were purposefully trying to hurt me by walking into my place of employment, announcing they were from the Board of Dentistry, and wanting to know where my home was, as if there was some sort of urgency. In my view, they were extremely unprofessional, as they had abused their power and didn't care who they hurt.

I recall the Dental Board putting out a newsletter in the state where I was trained, stating that over ninety percent of Board complaints could not be defended because of poor documentation. My response was: "Why are you telling us? We paid for an education, so why don't you send your newsletter to the school where we were trained?"

When I attended dental school, I was confused about documentation and went to several instructors for help. I recall none of them answered my questions or helped me in any way to better understand it. This tells me they didn't know how to do it either! I went on to my practice with no real skill in how to properly document... until I learned the hard way. Bottom line: to avoid a board complaint and/or a malpractice incident, write down *everything*! If it isn't written, it didn't happen. Period.

I went on and spent years researching and studying how to properly document *after* graduating from dental school. Since then, I've trained several dental offices on how to document patient charts to avoid risk. For those of you who don't understand what I mean, let me explain. Whenever a patient calls a dental office, presents for treatment, cancels, or fails an appointment, it's supposed to be documented. Whenever I address a group of dental professionals on this topic, I know that *maybe* eight to ten percent of those responsible for documentation have adequate skills to avert a dental board complaint or malpractice claim.

Since I've experienced what can happen when you are not trained to properly document your patient's chart, this is especially frightening to me. (No, I have never been the subject of a documented lawsuit.) Unless you've been in this situation, you have no idea how debilitating this can become and how it can turn your life upside down. A word to the wise: learning how to properly document is as important as learning how to prepare the perfect crown. Trust me on this.

I know my alma mater has since resolved this issue, but that doesn't change the disruption of someone's life and practice of those dental professionals who endured a malpractice suit or a grueling investigation by the Board of Dentistry. My friends and colleagues who have experienced the wrath of the Board agree: according to the Board, you are guilty until proven innocent.

I also hear administrative staff report that they have no time to document a failed or last-minute cancellation. Stop it. Today we have digital programs giving us immediate access to patient charts. How else are you going to defend your doctor from the patient who has consistently canceled appointments and then sues you because you didn't treat their severely decayed tooth?

Many patients "forget" about the treatment they need until it becomes an emergency. I've also experienced a patient's refusal to sign a treatment plan. Reminder: no signature on the treatment plan, no treatment. Patients back off when we can read them the dates they didn't show up, or when we can read notes from a treatment plan presentation concerning something they claim we never told them. This is what is meant by "an ounce of prevention is worth a pound of cure."

Also highly recommended is an annual review of the office policies around this topic. No one needs to have their life turned upside down because of a Board complaint or a malpractice suit (no matter how frivolous) they cannot defend.

CHAPTER ELEVEN

DENTAL INSURANCE
(and, Insurance Write-Offs)

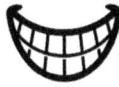

This happens to be one of my very favorite subjects. When I was a practicing dental hygienist, dental insurance was in its infancy; today, they boast as million-dollar companies. Just drive down any freeway in America, pick out the biggest, most beautiful building you can find, and I guarantee you it's an insurance company – with dental insurance policies for sale. Let's get real and talk the plain truth about dental insurance companies and dental insurance policies.

You might be surprised to learn about the origins of dental insurance: it was added to employee benefit packages roughly sixty-eight years ago to attract people to jobs. The maximums gradually rose to one thousand dollars or the extremely rare fifteen hundred dollars; however, while premiums continued to skyrocket over the years, the maximums have remained stagnant. In fact, one consultant explained to me that a thousand dollars is equal to less than one hundred thirty-five dollars today. So, what does this mean?? Here's what a dental practice in Chicago wrote:

> Unlike medical insurance, dental insurance is a fairly recent phenomenon. Dental insurance was first introduced in California in 1954, and quickly rose in popularity. By the 1970s, these plans were widely available and usually provided a maximum annual coverage of about $1000, **which is still about the maximum today**. The first plans established usual and customary rates for the area, and would typically pay 100% of preventative care, 80% of minor dental work, such as fillings, and 50% of major work, like crowns, and bridges.
>
> In the 70s, there grew another type of plan: the Dental Preferred Provider Organization, or PPO. The way these new plans worked is that in-network providers agreed to reduce their fees to offer treatment, and out-of-network providers would accept the insurance benefits and, patients would have to pay the difference between the provider's prices reduced fees and the insurance payments. PPO plans peaked in about 2011 with 65% market share, but have been losing ground ever since. New insurance plans are offering lower and lower payouts, and dentists are dropping out of the networks – unable to run a business on the low payout.[4]

---

[4] The History of Dental Insurance. (2015, Dec. 8). Wrigley Dental. https://www.wrigleyvilledental.com/blog/the-history-of-dental-insurance/

Clearly, dental insurance is NOT designed to get you healthy. Think about it. With the staggering incidence of dental disease being treated today, how can a thousand to fifteen hundred dollars a year make your mouth healthy? The average cost of a crown is approximately between $900 and $2,500 or more, so if your dental insurance company pays for fifty percent of that crown, one-third to one-half of your yearly benefit is used up…gone! Two cleanings (recommended for the healthiest mouth), fluoride treatment, two exams, some x-rays (yes, once a year), and two fillings, and your benefits are all used up.

Now let's consider the unhealthy mouth, the average condition of the average population. Since most people don't floss their teeth and since most dental disease occurs between your teeth, you are more than likely going to need more work than what is indicated above. So, how can your dental insurance even remotely keep you healthy? The intelligent answer is (drumroll, please) **Floss your teeth!** I am NOT being rude and please don't whine when your dentist sits you down and having diagnosed complete care, gives you a five-digit treatment plan!

The first thing out of your mouth is a question about how much your "insurance" covers, isn't it? Well, stop!! It's your dentist's job to diagnose complete care – to fully inform you of what state of health *or* disrepair your mouth is in from your dental exam. To fail and fully inform you is considered malpractice and, admit it, you'd be the first to sue the poor slob if there was something wrong that they missed or neglected to tell you!

If you have periodontal disease, the cost can be *huge* – but again, your dentist did not create this problem…YOU did. I've already explained that periodontal disease plays a role in the control of blood sugar in diabetes, high blood pressure, low birthweight in newborns, and many other medically compromising diseases. Therefore, it needs to be treated... hello-oh...did you hear me...*IT NEEDS TO BE TREATED!* And you don't ever rid yourself of periodontal disease, you only control it through your own efforts and four – yes, I said *four* – visits to your dental hygienist a year. Some dental insurance companies are now covering these visits in a more appropriate fashion, but it chews up your benefits fast. Why not do your part and prevent it altogether? Wow, what a concept.

Now I agree, our school systems do far too little to educate children about the prevention of dental disease. Instead, we backstroke with problems such as access to care, like it's some inevitable disease that instead of preventing, we need to find alternative methods to it clean up. Good grief – why not spend some money trying to prevent it or at the very least REDUCE ITS PREVALENCE in the first place?

I spoke to the Dental Director in one state about improving preventive dental education. This guy told me that "education doesn't work." Although I vehemently disagree, that was the approach this state took, and they are certainly still in the backstroke mode today.

I'm sorry, but education does work, information is valuable; cutting dental disease in half would put us well beyond the problem of access to care. *I'll say it again: there are no socioeconomic barriers to having a toothbrush and dental floss.* I swear, smokers spend more time having a smoke than they do cleaning their mouths. I know, this is human nature, but then *stop* whining about your dental bill because it's not our fault.

Let's talk about the details of your dental benefits plan. Why do you all get so angry when you receive your dental bill and find out that your dentist performed a procedure that your plan didn't cover? When we do something like an "indirect pulp cap." *it's because we need to!* If you have a deep decay in a tooth and it goes all the way down to the roof of your nerve, artery, and vein (termed the pulp chamber) we place a chemical or "medicine" to help protect the vitality of the tooth. If your tooth died because we *didn't* do it (And doing it doesn't guarantee anything, but it sure as hell gives you a fighting chance!) you'd be the first to blame us for its demise. OMG... we cannot win!

Let's get something straight: YOU can research your own damned insurance...PLEASE! Why is it you believe we should do all the work for you? More and more offices today have employees that do nothing but handle insurance, estimates, and appeals to denied claims. However, this costs the practice more money and, like any other business, the cost is passed along to the consumer. A business? Yes, just like the company you work for, a dental practice is a business where people come to work in a profession they have been trained to do, they make money, and it provides their family with an income. Duh.

And why do you all (okay, not all, but a lot of you) go around making moronic statements like: "All dentists are crooks; they just want to take your money." I would LOVE to put the next person I hear saying that in my shoes (or any of my colleagues' shoes) for just one week. Trust me; you'd be begging to go back to your own profession. We work hard – extremely hard – and we wear many, many hats; the average person couldn't do what we do day after day. I'm sure you've heard that the suicide rate for dentists is remarkably high, amongst the highest of any profession. Most people think it's because we work in tiny little spaces…ha! That's a ridiculously small part of it, no pun intended.

As I've stated, insurance companies are in the business of making money. Period. They determine the "usual and customary fee" for any service. Should a dentist sign on to these insurance companies, the dentist takes what is called a "write-off." What does that mean? Let me explain:

Instead of receiving our full fee, the fees we've established on our fee schedule, the insurance company decreases that fee and then pays the dental practice 50, 80, or 100% depending on the procedure. If the dentist agrees, he or she is taking a write-off. Over years in practice this can add up to tens of thousands of dollars. I looked at my "write-offs" one year and they were a staggering *fifty-five thousand dollars*! Heartbreaking for the demanding work we do.

So, when you make statements like, "I don't go to the dentist because I don't have insurance," we want to drop- kick you into next week…***you do not need dental insurance to go to the dentist!!*** And for those of you who do get insurance through your employer, we take a hit every time we treat you.

Speaking to both patients with, and without dental insurance, when you have an issue, stop hiding your head in the sand. At the very least, find out what is wrong and what you must do for it to remain stable until you can save the funds required to get it fully fixed. That's not rocket science. Waiting because "it stopped hurting" eventually makes it hurt more, will take longer to fix, and it will cost more.

Oh, and for the record: next time you get mad because your insurance didn't cover something you had done at your dentist, talk to your employer. They're the ones who negotiated your benefits package – dentists don't have anything to do with it – so put your dissatisfaction where it belongs.

CHAPTER TWELVE

THE OTHER DENTAL "INSURANCE"

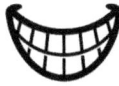

N ow that we've covered traditional dental insurance – it's time to get crystal clear on a different kind of "insurance" that isn't actually insurance at all. What is it? It's welfare, state aid, and medical assistance programs. You are aware people abuse the system, right? You bet they do, costing taxpayers millions of dollars a year.

Let's be clear on one point: there are people using state aid dental coverage who really need and deserve it: single mothers, the disabled, veterans, the mentally incapacitated, and low-income children – they are the ones the system is designed to protect. However, there are also able-bodied individuals who cheat, lie, and take advantage – and I can tell you straight up: these are the patients who cause most of the problems in any low-income facility. They behave as if they are entitled, and they are the first to complain when a procedure isn't covered.

These people walk in wearing hundred-dollar shoes, designer jeans, and purses; they're talking on iPhones (that they got on state aid!), they smoke (a costly habit!), and have manicured nails and highlighted hair, yet many haven't brushed their teeth for days and, what's more, often cop an attitude. I personally have no time in my busy schedule for these individuals and I don't care if their teeth hurt or not. If they can afford all the above, they can take care of their own dental issues. I fault the states for not looking more closely at these deadbeats for the astronomical amounts they are costing this country.

Some welfare recipients get angry because what they call "insurance" won't pay for crowns, root canal treatments on back teeth, or gum disease. I want to ask them, "Seriously, you're mad because my taxes pay for your care, I do the work at no charge to you, and you're mad?" WOW! Some of these patients will pay for their own crowns and bridges, then turn around and say, "My insurance can pay for the fillings." I want to go into my office and scream, "Loser!!" Sweetheart, if you can pay for your crowns, you can pay for it all!

I have a GREAT idea: let's dole out free dental care ONLY for those patients who financially qualify and can demonstrate outstanding home care, responsibility around keeping their appointments, and respecting the privilege they've been given. How about drug testing? After all, if you can afford drugs, you can certainly afford to pay for your dental care.

Putting some of this in order might just save the taxpayers some money, or perhaps this savings could go towards our educational system. As the saying goes, kids are our future, yet the English language is so poorly taught today it makes my skin crawl. Stop the dental freeloaders and put that money to better use.

The dentist would make a great gatekeeper and if you present with a filthy mouth (and we can tell if you cleaned up just for your appointment today, friend) your *free* care is denied, period. Oh, and people who make appointments and then don't show? Three strikes and *free* dental care is denied – permanently. How about dentists watching for suspicious indications that patients are abusing the system…perhaps a suitable time to have them investigated. And for sure, when parents don't show for their children's appointments more than twice, those kids should be moved to foster care as there are certainly other issues being neglected as well.

I received a copy of a letter from a colleague who worked in a facility that was funded by state and federal governments. This letter was certainly an eye-opener. After almost six years in one of these facilities, the author saw an article in a local paper indicating that this state was asking for federal aid to fund their healthcare. It gives an example of what can be seen in one of these facilities, so I've included it here.

To Whom This May Concern:

I have been thinking about writing this letter for a long time. After reading an article sent to me by a friend, and hearing the complaints from colleagues in medicine and dentistry, I've decided to get it done. I'm beyond disgusted with what's happening in this country, as well as in this state! I will not tell you who I am as I need to protect my income, but suffice it to say, this country is in the toilet. I was born in the '50s, raised in the '60s, survived the '70s and was educated in the '80s. 2016 looks exceptionally bad as I watch how this once great country has changed, and not for the better.

I simply want to share with you that I have seen as a large contributor to what is destroying our Land of the Free. I was encouraged to hear the President say he was going to put Americans back to work. Then I said out loud, "What about those who don't want to work at anything but working the system?" I'm told a supervisor once said, "It's not our job to discern who's cheating and who isn't cheating." Sorry, I wholeheartedly disagree; until someone stands up and exposes these cheaters, the swamp will continue to fill with sewage.

I work in the health industry that deals with people on state aid; what I have personally witnessed over the past several years is positively appalling, I must tell you how ridiculous this government of ours has become. Here is what I've seen:

1. People on state aid driving a Porsche, new Cadillac, BMWs...BRAND NEW CARS OF EVERY TYPE ENTERING OUR FACILITY!

2. With *very* few exceptions, women come in with their fingernails and toenails done, their hair professionally colored and they come in late because they wanted to sleep in (Boo-hoo, they DON'T WORK.) I've heard staff members state that they "want to go on state aid so they can get their nails done regularly."

3. One young lady came in to get treatment and the girls noticed her cute jeans. They asked her where she got them. No surprise...they were $185 designer jeans.

Once again, she was receiving FREE TREATMENT ON STATE AID.

4. I've heard of vacations, the likes of which I've never taken: "We're spending the winter in the Cayman Islands…" Yup…getting free treatment. How about going to the East Coast for the summer? I think that would be nice, but I've never done it…I WORK!

5. "I'm going to Peru for a month…will my treatment be completed by then?" I asked her, "How do you afford a month in Peru if you're on state aid?" Answer: "I work three jobs" Question: "How do you qualify for state aid if you are working three jobs?" Answer: "I get paid on two of my jobs 'under the table.' Question: "Isn't that cheating the system?" NO ANSWER.

6. One of our clients has two of his kids in private school and they're receiving state aid.

7. I've seen a man purchase $10,000 CASH worth of irrigation pipe for his "grow" and turn around and buy the child with him an ice cream with food stamps. I wanted to slap him. It was blatant.

8. I've personally witnessed people who have come to this state *just* to get their medical/dental done "for free" and they proudly report they own a house, on a lake in Texas.

9. Designer purses, Ray-Ban sunglasses, and designer glasses…it goes on and on.

10. I met one woman who got a job, but she quit. She made more money on the system than she could working.

11. I keep seeing driver's licenses from other states and on our state aid. Then I ask: "Oh, did you just move here?" Answer: "No, I've been here for about three-and-a-half years." REALLY?! How are these people qualifying for state aid?

12. Just last week a young mother came in for treatment and she was texting the father of her baby, apologizing for having spent $100 on make-up. She went on to text: "but that money could have gone to diapers." He responded that state aid should pay for diapers, because he understood how important make-up was to her. Really?? A staff member saw this in a colleague's office.

13. Another patient said she and the father of her three children don't marry because he makes over $100,000 and then they wouldn't qualify for state aid.

14. People come to this state during trimming season (trimming marijuana) and make anywhere from $25-$28/hr. cash. A pharmacist reported that they can cut themselves, go to the ER for treatment, tell the hospital, "I *just* moved here and I'm staying with a friend while I look for permanent residence." They're put on an "open card," get free treatment, free meds, and within a few weeks are assigned to a medical and dental clinic for free treatment. *They don't live here, and they make enough money to pay for the injury themselves!*

15. One of my friend's assistants did a working interview in a periodontal clinic and saw a welfare patient (from the office where she was full-time employed) getting an

estimate for seven implants. She'd already presented to the state aid clinic with five implants.

16. Another patient on state aid showed off her new infant, proudly reporting that it had taken four in-vitro tries to get pregnant.

What the hell is going on here? This is ludicrous, ridiculous, and embarrassing. Instead of worrying about more taxes, why not start scouting these cheaters? Disability insurance companies do. You'd save millions! How about just starting with *requiring a valid driver's license?*

These patients also display an outrageous list of inappropriate behavior and comments:

1. They fail confirmed appointments over and over and over. Then when they have a toothache and an emergency, they whine and complain about having to sit and wait.

2. They get incredibly rude and annoyed about having to fill out the required paperwork.

3. They come in stoned and having consumed alcohol and get volatile when we refuse treatment.

4. They display an incredible sense of entitlement.

5. They complain (and I mean loudly) that their "insurance" doesn't pay for enough. Their lack of understanding how money works reveals their lack of education and their stupidity.

6. One patient on state aid was told he needed three crowns, but was informed that state aid didn't pay

for laboratory-constructed crowns. His comment was rude and revealing: "I don't think you should assume I can't afford three $995.00 crowns just because I'm on state aid." My dentist friend told me he almost bit off his tongue; he wanted to say: "If you can afford three crowns, you can afford everything else on this treatment plan." He went on to say:

- *How about urine testing? You do drugs, NO state aid!*
- *How about a limited time to receive state aid? Give them two years to get their head together and get a job, then they're done. Some of these participants have two and three generations that have collected state aid.*
- *How about requiring a valid driver's license?*
- *How about setting up some rules, regulations, and guidelines, huh? If you've got them, we've NEVER seen them enforced!*

Then you have the audacity to call my social security an entitlement...REALLY?! I've worked my entire life and that means fifty-plus years of contributing to our society and the forward movement of this country. Furthermore, I've earned the right to vote...if you don't pay Uncle Sam, you don't vote. If you don't work and pay taxes, YOU DON'T GET TAX RETURNS, NO MATTER HOW MANY CHILDREN YOU HAVE.

Why does this state and this country keep giving everything away? I, along with my brother and sister, was raised by a single mom. She didn't go on welfare, which by the way was what it was called, not some fancy name to hide the fact that it's WELFARE. She WORKED! She worked long and hard and made my sister's Easter dresses out of old curtains. We drank powdered milk and ate lots of chicken. State aid recipients walk in with their Starbucks…with no shame. Oh, and by the way… food stamps pay for Starbucks. (I know this because a friend of mine works there.) Yes…a mocha latte is covered by welfare recipients, paid for by you, whichever way you prefer looking at it.

Sincerely, moving to a state with some backbone (i.e., tell them to get a job) would make me feel a lot better. Some states don't deserve any federal funding because they do nothing to help themselves. There are paid government employees who are giving away money to people who sincerely don't deserve it. They need to lose their jobs and replace them with hard-working investigators who won't suck the breast of our government just for a paycheck.

He signed it, "Fed Up with This State's Welfare System!"

CHAPTER THIRTEEN

ENTER DENTAL MEMBERSHIPS

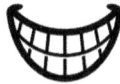

I've yet to meet a dental practice owner who loves dealing with dental insurance companies. As I look back on my dental practice, these companies caused more problems than they solved. Today, I tell dental practices how important it is to educate patients in the truth that:

> Dental Insurance Companies are not designed
> to make your patients healthy ~ they're designed to
> make themselves wealthy!

I often thought I'd be far happier if I eliminated them, but then how could I successfully retain patients?

Today, there's a solution and I'm excited to talk about it! Have you heard of dental memberships? Let me introduce you to this amazing concept designed for those patients who don't have dental insurance:

The dental patient first pays a registration fee to be part of the program, then pays a negligible monthly fee, offering them access to a list of procedures they otherwise might avoid. Again, I can't tell you how many times I've heard someone say they can't go to the dentist because they don't have dental insurance. This is simply not the case! Those who do have insurance are sick of the denials, rising premiums, and less coverage. Let's eliminate all the drama, drop the insurance plans, and get patients signed up for a Dental Membership Plan! Once you are part of a plan, here are the immediate advantages to maintaining your dental health:

- You can confidently get your regular check-ups without having to be certain it's been *exactly* six months since your last check-up. Some dental insurance plans won't pay for a check-up if you aren't exactly six months or more past your last cleaning and check-up. I've seen insurance companies deny a claim when the patient got their check-up *one day* short of six months. That's petty!

- You can agree to treatment without waiting for approval, on which dental insurance companies have been known to drag their feet. Some dental treatment can't wait!

- You can move forward with a treatment plan designed for your dental health, doing procedures not covered by a dental insurance plan.

This is a no-brainer and I'm surprised someone didn't come up with it sooner! I certainly would have signed on.

CHAPTER FOURTEEN

DENTAL CONSULTANTS

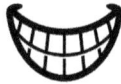

T hroughout this book I've spoken about my life as a dentist; what you may not know is that I currently own a staffing job board, and for that reason I attend many types of dental conventions as a vendor. I cannot tell you how many people approach my booth stating they are consultants. Dental consultants come in all shapes and sizes, and I know that ninety-nine percent of them are what I call wannabes. Indeed, most of these "consultants" haven't even been breathing long enough to have the kind of experience necessary to demand the salary of a dental consultation.

I know that today there are many great consultants and consulting firms. I know this because I research what they do while considering whether my staffing company may want to partner with them. The ones I've researched can truly solve any problem you can hand them. I often find myself asking them, "where were you when I was in private practice?"

Years ago, I hired way more consultants than I'd like to admit, and I wish I had just a small percentage of that money back.

If I'd spent it on leadership courses, psychotherapy – anything but consultants – I'd have been much farther ahead. It's simply my opinion, but when you hire a consultant and they never set foot in your office or ask to see your numbers, how can they possibly know where the problems lie or what needs to be done about them?

There is, however, one tip I learned from a consultant that was extremely beneficial: always, always, always present complete care. This means doing a highly involved and thorough exam on the patient's first visit that includes determining the patient's personal dental goals and presenting all care that is deemed necessary. This allows them to decide what they will or will not do – then, if the patient decides to forego care, there's no liability.

That same consultant recommended that we ("we" being the eight dental practices present at the meeting) stop taking payment from a particular large and powerful insurance company. We were instructed to print out the insurance form, place it in a self-addressed, stamped envelope and have the patient mail it. Too often insurance companies tell us they "never received the claim" – and all too often, patients believe them.

The patient then receives the payment and takes the hit of the write-off. Furthermore, if the patient mails the form, and the insurance company claims they never received it, that excuse becomes moot. You can believe it or not, but I've been to meetings where the speaker, having been a former employee of a dental insurance company, told us every eighth claim is shredded. When the patient mails the claim, we stop looking inept.

I've already told you that dental insurance companies *always* write off a portion of the dentist's fee, and that early in my private practice I lost fifty-five thousand dollars to them. Now, I found that to be a tremendous loss, especially since I had a small practice, so I took the consultant's recommendation and ran with it. Here's the deal:

1. The patient pays the full amount of treatment at the time of the appointment.
2. They mail the insurance form we've provided; it will be stamped and addressed.
3. They wait for their insurance to pay them, so the dental practice gets paid in full and the patient takes the loss (write-off).
4. Most patients are not going to agree to this and will find a dental practice that will take their insurance, forcing the practice to take the hit.

If you're a layperson and thinking, *You guys make so much money, and charge too much, why does it matter?*, go back and read the earlier chapters on the time and financial commitments involved in becoming a dentist, as well as the overhead we carry. In the meantime, let's take a look at what happened to the practices who took the advice of the consultant.

- One practice was in a financial position to do it, so it worked for them.
- One practice lost half of their patients.
- One practice went bankrupt.
- Five offices didn't do it!

I was the practice who lost half of her patients. Fortunately for me, I'd been doing a lot of cosmetic dentistry, which is not covered by insurance. It still hurt deeply to have my friends and family leave my practice over dental insurance.

The moral of this story: when a consultant recommends a dental practice stop accepting insurance payments, (requiring the patient to pay the bill), you better be sure you have a strong following and that you can afford to lose revenue because patients (including your own family and friends) will leave your practice.

It is my belief that no consultant should be making any such suggestion without presenting a method to determine if the practice involved can afford to risk such a move.

CHAPTER FIFTEEN

FLUORIDE

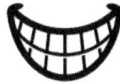

I will forever be in the dark about the bad attitude concerning water fluoridation. I'm not certain what the issues are regarding fluoride, but I can tell you, except for enamel fluorosis, I have not seen an increase in any disease from the fluoridation of a water supply. Some say fluoride is a poison, and it is *if you ingest too much*, but we can say that about a lot of things that are beneficial in normal amounts – including water!

I was born in a state where in 1955 fluoride was placed in the water at one part/million. Today there are thirty-, forty- and fifty-year-old individuals I saw in my practice who had no or minimal tooth decay. Then, having gone to work in a neighboring state where there was no water fluoridation, the decay I saw, especially in children, was heartbreaking.

That brings me to a job I took in a state where there was no water fluoridation coupled with extremely poor nutrition, and what I saw was inexcusable. Parents would bring their kids in carrying soda and bags of candy, and their oral health reflected this. I saw one ten-year-old child with every tooth decayed to the gumline! This was the only time I ever contacted child protective services and to date, I'm not sure the child was ever removed to a more supportive environment.

These young patients prompted me to call and speak to the Chief Dental Officer at the state capital. After a short conversation where I asked about the state's lack of water fluoridation and education regarding better nutrition, and as I told you earlier, he coolly stated, "Education doesn't work," and bade me farewell.

Another idiotic bureaucrat collecting a paycheck supplied by your taxes.

I went to dental school in the same fluoridated state in which I was raised. We attended lectures ad nauseam regarding the biochemistry and efficacy of fluoride and water fluoridation. In some instances, as we entered the lecture hall and the professor was stating the lecture was going to be on fluoride, you'd see students turning around and leaving. All we cared about was that it worked to prevent tooth decay, causes no medical problems, can be adjusted where we see enamel fluorosis and, in the right concentration, is safe.

At some point the water fluoridation in my state was changed from one part/million to .7 parts/million, when it was determined that one part/million was creating some enamel fluorosis in children. Today, enamel fluorosis can be successfully "bleached" by any number of products that keep the "bleach" in close proximity to the tooth structure for a brief period and on a regular basis.

Fluorine and chlorine sit side by side on the periodic table. There's chlorine in our water supply to prevent bacterial growth and no one objects to it other than, depending on the concentration, it doesn't taste or smell particularly good right out of the faucet.

A fun story sent to me by a colleague who knew I was looking for Down In the Mouth material.

I was working in a clinic where patients were seen on a state aid program. After doing an exam on a young child with her father sitting in the room, I gave the go-ahead to have my assistant clean her teeth and apply fluoride. Her father angrily responded with, "No fluoride!"

Curious, I asked why he was so adamant about this, to which he replied that fluoride was a poison, and he didn't want his child exposed to it. I looked at him and calmly said, "Much like those cigarettes sticking out of your pocket?" I could only assume he smoked in the house and in his car, because I could smell cigarettes on my young patient! Ignorance is bliss!

CHAPTER SIXTEEN

THE OTHER "F" WORD (WHAT ARE YOUR EXPECTATIONS?)

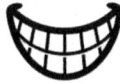

I have a dear friend who spent a ton of money on orthodontic treatment (braces). I think he may have even gotten them twice. When I asked him if he was flossing, he replied, "No, I don't, because I have fixed retainers." He went on to say he eats very well (and he really does focus on his diet), he brushes well, and furthermore, he doesn't consume sugar. (Which saved me from having to tell him about the outrageous amount of sugar that's found in processed foods.)

The point is, he didn't feel he needed to floss, that his healthy lifestyle insulated him from dental disease. I explained that all of his healthy habits did help, but if he didn't floss the garbage out from between his teeth, eventually he was going to have some degree of dental disease. The bacteria are there, and they will thrive, irrespective of diet! I ended the conversation by recommending super floss to get under those retainers. Nothing else was going to make a significant difference.

The reason I tell this story is because many patients balk about being presented with an expensive treatment plan when they won't floss and don't brush properly. What do they expect? I also mention this because I know a lot of dental professionals simply tell their patients they "need to floss," without telling them *why* they need to floss. I'm not certain what type of behavioral change they're expecting, but I'd bet the percentage of patients who change their habits is negligible. I can't tell you how many patients (and dental assistants) have told me I explain flossing in a manner that makes sense and they've started doing it as a result.

You can't fully expect a good check-up without regular flossing. Why? Because when you don't, *forty percent* of your tooth structure isn't being cleaned. Bacteria is a nasty colony of tenacious goo that needs to be mechanically interrupted/removed, and no brush (yes, even "electric" ones) and no mouthwash will get between your teeth to do it. So, if you choose to forego flossing, change your expectations, because eventually it's going catch up with you! This I can promise.

Chapter Seventeen

DENTAL SCHOOL DIDN'T PREPARE ME TO BE YOUR BANKER OR YOUR BABYSITTER

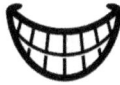

or years I would treat a patient and hear, "I'll pay my bill once the insurance has paid" – this was customary practice back then. The insurance company was supposed to pay the claim within thirty days, but many times they were denied and fell into the appeals process. By the time the claim was paid, and the patient took care of their portion, the dentist had been waiting up to ninety days or longer. As a result, I often found myself carrying a hefty accounts receivable. (For those who don't know what that means, its money owed for services already rendered.) Not surprisingly, this makes it rather difficult to successfully run a business.

Today, software programs can immediately determine the patient's portion of the claim and they are expected to pay their portion in full following treatment. Also, there are companies that will lend funds for dental treatment (as well as veterinary, elective medical, and chiropractic treatments); however, one must be a good credit risk and interest rates can be quite high.

Still, there are issues with receiving timely payment. Remember the story from Chapter 2, where the woman told her young daughter they wouldn't be able to get a Christmas tree because they had to pay their copay? While this is an extreme example of rudeness, the occurrence is not as unusual as you might think. You don't walk into the local grocery store, fill your cart with food, and then tell the cashier, "Bill me." And if your boss announced you had to wait for your paycheck until HR had a chance to evaluate your work, you'd likely object or quit. So why do you think it's okay for us to wait for our paycheck?

Another issue that continues to occur (and makes me nuts) is patients bringing their small children with them to their appointments. *We are dental care providers, not babysitters.* It's as if patients think the team can stop whatever they're doing for an hour to watch their kids! Really? I had one patient set her infant's carrier in the hall while she went into a room, out of eyeshot of her child, to have her x-rays taken! Who does that?

How about the woman who insisted she bring the baby stroller into the small dental hygiene operatory so she could rock it while she had her teeth cleaned? Then, when the baby started crying, she had to be sat up so she could hold her child until he fell asleep again. No dental hygienist should be expected to do a decent job while putting up with that type of behavior.

Know this, I'm just barely touching on what I've seen and heard. I could go on for chapters. My assistant even suggested I post on Facebook and ask my colleagues to send me their outrageous stories. No thanks. I envisioned an eighteen-wheeler backing onto my property and dumping a mountain of letters.

There is the legal liability providers can incur if a child gets injured in their office. I cannot fathom what crosses the minds of people who let their children loose in the office and expect we will watch them. How rude, stupid, and irresponsible! They can get into dangerous areas of the clinic, walk into equipment, and touch things they shouldn't be touching. I suspect those parents would also be the first to sue if the child did get hurt...enough said!

People: get yourself a babysitter or reschedule your appointment. We have work to do.

CHAPTER EIGHTEEN

PARENTS, YOU NEED TO BE QUIET... REALLY, JUST SHUT UP!

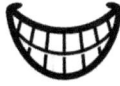

There were no beautiful dental practices in the suburbs where I grew up. When my siblings and I had a dental appointment, Mom would drive us downtown and drop us off at the Medical Arts Building, saying: "Go inside, sit down and be quiet until you're called back to see the dentist." Then she'd go shopping and pick us up an hour later.

Oh, how times have changed.

Today, in most states, you can't just leave your kids at the dentist and go about your business. A parent or a legal guardian must be present, especially if an irreversible procedure is to take place in a dental office. If the person accompanying the child is not a legal guardian, a signed permission slip by said guardian is required. There are also informed consents to sign and questions to be asked and answered.

Then there is the other extreme: the so-called helicopter parents who insist on coming into the exam room with their kids. They hover over their child before and during the procedure; they make statements like, "It's not going to hurt" or "You're going to get a shot." Stupid! Stupid, stupid. Are you aware that your words and behavior are transferring your fear and your issues to your child? Jeez, people, just shut up and sit down. You are here to observe, not participate. I've been doing this longer than you've been breathing. I got this!

I worked in a clinic where the doctor/owner would not allow parents to come back with their children. His theory was, "If you don't trust me to treat your child appropriately, then you need a different dental practice." That was a great rule! Let me tell you why.

Children learn their fear of the dentist from their parents running their mouths about their own experiences. They use words like "hurt," "shot," and "pain." They discuss their own fears out loud, at home, in front of their kids, and those very same children learn to be fearful!

These parents are also distracting; their constant hovering and talking divides the dentist's focus, decreases their control, and interferes with treatment. In short, they become a liability. My very mild-mannered colleague/friend put it so clearly when a father kept saying to his son, "It's going to be alright" and "Try to relax."

"Sir," he said in a very terse tone, "in this room, I'm in charge."

You need to get this, parents. You are not doing your children any favors; you are actually making them afraid and jeopardizing the success of the procedure. If you want to be in the room, sit down, be quiet and observe.

If you truly want to be a supportive parent, speak positively about going to the dentist. Try to make it a fun experience, because that's what we try to do for the kiddos. And, for your child's sake, make oral care a habit by starting them young. I have an acquaintance who is terrified of the dentist and has *never* taken her thirteen-year-old. She has transferred all her fear to her daughter to carry for the remainder of her life. Sorry, but again, that's ignorance, and the antithesis of good parenting!

The parents I applaud walk their kids back, get them situated, and tell them they'll be right outside waiting for them to be done. This teaches them: 1) going to the dentist is "what we do"; 2) how to become independent; and 3) self-esteem.

Parents, this bears repeating: if you are allowed to go back with your kiddo, and you intend to stay, SIT DOWN AND BE QUIET!

CHAPTER NINETEEN

TELEVISION COMMERCIALS

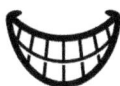

I'm not certain where I got the idea that television commercials were supposed to be truthful, but when I got some dental experience under my belt, I started noticing that they were anything but. It's a matter of knowledge and really paying attention to their claims.

Early on in my career I accepted an invitation to do a blind interview by a company that was researching some dental products. I was asked if I had heard of the commercial advertising a product that was supposed to kill germs and stop bad breath. The commercial showed something (I'm not sure what because these bacteria are microscopic) going down the drain in a white sink! I told them that I had indeed seen the commercial and was asked for my opinion.

I replied that a good stiff martini would kill those free-floating bacteria that *could* mature and organize, causing bad breath. I elaborated on this, saying that if they were being a hundred percent truthful, they would explain that this product did nothing to affect the organized bacterial plaque that is stuck between your teeth, under the gumline. In fact, no mouthwash could reach the bacteria that *are* causing bad breath.

The interview ended, and I was never asked again.

How about the television commercial with the dentist reporting that she's worried about her patients who have tooth and gum sensitivity? Malarky! Tooth and gum sensitivity aren't even on the list of issues dentists deal with daily. All she'd have to do is make a recommendation to help curb the problem; it certainly doesn't keep her up at night!

Oh, and did you know that you can brush and floss at the same time… NOT! Effective plaque removal is a site-specific endeavor that takes about four to five minutes twice a day. You smokers spend more time smoking cigarettes through-out the day. You nonsmokers spend more time texting. Even when you use a Waterpik, you must pause between each tooth, inside and outside, to be effective.

Let's talk about the movie star that says she's embracing getting older, and then she mumbles something about getting "gum issues due to aging." This is another nonsensical excuse for getting bad gums and losing their teeth. I am seventy years old, and I have all my teeth. I did lose four premolars when I got braces and I did have my "wisdom" teeth removed. (I don't know why they call them "wisdom" teeth; you get them at eighteen and you have zero wisdom at that age.)

My gums are pink, stippled, and knife-edged (all good things), and I repeat: *I am seventy years old!* Furthermore, the advertised toothpaste has never touched my mouth, as has no other "special" toothpaste. I simply floss and brush my teeth regularly and thoroughly. If you want what I have, stop being lazy, and just do it!

There's a toothbrush commercial that I have seen but can't tell you what is being said because I'm simply noting the sub-liminal message. It's a toothbrush that appears to be removing debris from the cheek side of the teeth and the tongue side of the teeth *at the same time*. I've even questioned patients about what that commercial is telling them and consistently they report what the visual portrays. Then I must be the bearer of bad (and obvious) news: it is physically impossible for a tooth-brush to do this. Period.

"It also works on crowns, veneers, and dentures!" – that's the tooth whitening commercial. Fact: this product may remove any stains on the surface of these restorations, but it won't "whiten" them. They will forever be the color they were when they were placed. If they matched your teeth at that time and you are whitening now, your teeth will be whiter and brighter than the veneers and crowns.

This is a new one I just saw on some health website:

"Buy this dental tool and you'll never have to go to the dentist to get your teeth cleaned ever again!" The "before" picture is one of deeply stained teeth; the "after" photo shows a clean, bright white tooth surface. This is more than just a slap in the face of dental professionals, add a punch to the gut! Do you know how long it took me to get proficient at properly and thoroughly cleaning teeth? It took years, and my mentor was a periodontist (gum god!). To advertise that you can clean your teeth at home with this tool is reckless, not to mention dangerous.

First, although they give you a mouth mirror, learning how to work backward in a mirror is extremely difficult. Are you going to stop breathing long enough to clean the inside of your mouth so your mirror doesn't fog up?

Oh! And do you have any root exposure? If so, be careful because the roots are much softer than the crown of the tooth and you don't want to gouge the root surface. If you do gouge the root, that gives the oral microbes a wonderful place to adhere to and grow. The plaque is then out of the reach of dental floss, causing more disease over time.

Be careful of the soft tissue attachment! You don't know what I'm talking about? Hah – didn't think so! If you damage this attachment, it may not reattach properly, creating bigger problems than a chunk of tartar. (Hey, the proper term is calculus.) And don't forget the teeth in the back of your mouth – you know, the areas that are difficult, even for highly-trained dental professionals to clean. "But, oh yah, you have that handy-dandy tool!" said no dental hygienist ever.

Using this or any similar device would be the single worst dental health decision a patient can make. Think about it. You're not a licensed dental professional, so stop acting like what we do is so simple that anyone can do it.

And finally, there is a commercial so outrageous only a nut would try it. Ready? It's a commercial about *at- home teeth straightening.* Apparently, you are supposed to take your own impressions with material you receive in the mail. You send the impressions in, and you receive several trays worn at intervals that will straighten your teeth without stepping into a dental office.

I'm sorry, but OMG! Are you aware the candidates who apply for the specialty of Orthodontics are the crème de la crème of their dental class? They are the top dogs, people! The best and the brightest! When I graduated from dental school, the specialty of Orthodontics was the most difficult to get into. Personally, I hated the orthodontic courses – they were extremely difficult, and my talents were in reconstruction.

So, let's talk about some of the pitfalls of doing your own orthodontic treatment.

What if your issue is a bone growth problem and you need surgery to create enough room for the proper alignment required to "straighten" your teeth? Orthodontists take several radiographs to help determine their course of treatment.

What if you have periodontal disease and don't know it? That's potentially disastrous. You start moving teeth that are compromised with support issues and you'll end up with more problems than crooked teeth!

What if you have an ankylosed tooth? This is a tooth that has fused to bone and will not move. I've come up against these teeth and they are extremely difficult to remove, should that be necessary.

And take your own impression? Even I can't take impressions like an Orthodontic Assistant can. Don't even try to tell me a layperson can take an accurate impression that's going to determine their course of treatment!

These are just a couple of possible scenarios that could impact your plans for straighter teeth. Some of you will go ahead and do it anyway, but after having orthodontic treatment twice, I would say, no way! What you don't know *can* hurt you!

Suck it up, get to the dentist, and let them do the job they were trained to do.

Now I pay attention to commercials and advertisements I see; it's simply about sales and money. It appears that companies will say and do anything to sell their product. Consumer beware!

CHAPTER TWENTY

MYTHS DISPELLED

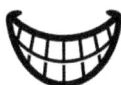

Okay, we're going to talk some real truths here, so sit back, be quiet and listen. The first is that when you tell us your ridiculous dental stories, know that as soon as we're back in the lab or in sterilization, we are laughing. Yes, laughing at you, and our inability to fathom how you could think we'd believe you. Here are just a few...

"When he took my tooth out, he actually had his knee up on my chest..."

Stop it, just stop. No one – and I mean *no* dental professional in the modern world – ever put his or her knee up on your chest to remove your tooth. You're assuming we literally "pull" teeth, when what we actually do is detach the soft tissue and elevate them. Can teeth be stubborn? Do we sometimes have to circumferentially remove a millimeter of crestal bone, rock the tooth cheek to tongue in order to stretch the ligamental fibers? Yes, but never a knee goes up on a chest. Sorry.

"My dentist told me I have a lot of cavities because my saliva is very acidic..."

You gotta be kidding, man! Have you never stopped to consider that we study – *in depth* – the biochemistry of saliva? Now, let's set the story straight:

Saliva has recuperative properties, meaning it has free-floating Ca+ and Ph ions. Saliva replenishes calcium and phosphorous lost to our teeth when we eat acidic fruit and drink carbonated beverages, or due to the acid production from bacteria. Furthermore, saliva neutralizes acid from these sources, helping slow the development of cavities. Saliva contains chemicals that begin the digestion of carbohydrates and fats. Once again, digestion begins in the mouth, due – along with chewing – to the biochemical nature of saliva.

So, when you come into our office, sit in our chair, and make moronic statements that some dentist told you your problem is one of acidic saliva, what you are really saying is, "I don't want to take personal responsibility for my dental condition." Nothing absolves you from having to pick up a toothbrush and dental floss and clean your teeth. Those types of statements just make you sound stupid, lazy, and irresponsible.

Quite recently I was told by an acquaintance that her mother was going to a new kind of "bio dentist." Apparently this is a new specialty of dentistry and he told her mother they consider "the whole body when practicing dentistry." As you have read on these pages, we're *supposed* to consider the "entire health of the patient when practicing dentistry." Her mother was told the notches at her gumline were from having "an acidic system." After several conversations with dental friends, and watching them shake their head, we've concluded they're likely what we call abfraction lesions. None of us, young and older, have ever heard of any such disorder called an "acidic system."

Oh, and by the way, if by some very remote possibility your dentist really did tell you your problem was acidic saliva, they are either not a licensed dentist (and therefore didn't pass boards) or they graduated from dental school prior to 1950 and shouldn't be practicing dentistry. Either way, I'd get a new dentist!

"I was told that my gum disease is inherited…"

NOT! In 99.9% of all cases, gum disease or what we call periodontal disease, is caused by uncontrolled growth and colonization of bacteria. Yes, there is one form of periodontal disease that is inherited; that form is called Juvenile Periodontitis, and it affects adolescents, not adults. By the time these patients reach adulthood their teeth are gone, so as an adult, the excuse of inheritance doesn't cut it. And by the way, in the thirty-eight years since I graduated from dental school, I've never met one patient with an inherited form of periodontal disease. Sounds as if it's exceedingly rare.

As infants, we are born with relatively bacteria-free mouths. We acquire the first oral bacteria as we pass through the birth canal, then, as the individual who's feeding us in infancy checks the temperature of our food. They typically check it with their upper lip prior to putting it in our mouths – thus, the inoculation of our mouths with their bacteria. Add kissing (people or pets), biting our nails, sharing drinks and food, and any other type of behavior involving our mouths, and there you have it. The bacteria, acquired over a series of human interactions, is now yours forever.

I'd be willing to bet some of you have even shared toothbrushes... again, transferring bacteria. If an individual with periodontal disease marries someone without periodontal bacteria, within five years, the latter individual will have acquired the bacteria of the spouse and, unless they control the growth of these bacteria, will eventually display some signs of the disease.

But there's good news! Though you never rid yourself of these disease-causing bugs, if you thoroughly clean your teeth (and I mean all five surfaces of every tooth, twice/day) and visit your dentist at the recommended intervals, you will not bear the cost and heartache of this disease. How do I know this to be so absolutely true? I am the offspring of a woman who lost several teeth to periodontal disease. *Her* mother lost *all* her teeth to the disease. I control the bacteria and the only teeth I've lost were third molars and the four premolars they took out when I had braces. They will lay me to rest with all remaining teeth and no disease.

Once again, it appears to us that *you* don't want to own the problem; you've got to find a way to defer blame, so you blame it on your genes, rather than taking charge of your home care and dental visits. Take my cousin, for example: as intelligent as he was, he told me his sister brushes, and flosses religiously and still has periodontal disease. No amount of conversation was going to change his mind.

Unfortunately, I think he left out the part about her heavy smoking habit and the fact she may have gotten religious about dental health when it was far too late. Once it's late in the game, everything must change to help control the disease and hang on to those teeth.

- no more smoking
- dental visits every three months (So many of you want to go every four months, but as I learned from an exceptional periodontist and my mentor, the late Dr. Patrick Gaspard, the bacteria that are most damaging are mature in ninety days.)
- exemplary home care, and all this with
- a high probability of periodontal surgery

And the smoking thing? Today, we all know smoking causes damage to our bodies. What it does to the body will also impact the mouth. Smoking affects our immune system and our body's ability to fight disease. Oral disease is no exception.

"I have soft teeth and I've had problems with my teeth since I was a kid…"

Ahhh, one of my personal favorites…the soft teeth excuse. There is no such thing as soft teeth unless you are one of the unfortunate individuals who have inherited Amelogenesis Imperfecta or Dentinogenesis Imperfecta. This means imperfectly formed enamel or dentin. Enamel is the outer portion of the tooth that covers the portion seen when you look in your mouth. Dentin is that part of the tooth that is under enamel (on the crown of the tooth) and under cementum (on the root of the tooth).

Dentin is what makes enamel strong. When a tooth breaks, in most cases, it's from tooth decay that has invaded dentin, undermining enamel, and causing it to break. In Dentinogenesis

Imperfecti, dentin doesn't form properly, and enamel breaks easily without the support of healthy dentin. Make no mistake: if you display either of these disorders it's apparent and easily identified. The patient will display other physical anomalies with either of these disorders, such as missing or minimal sweat glands, thin hair, and bone disorders, to name a few. This puts the soft teeth excuse in the toilet.

"I have bad teeth, just like my mom and dad, sister, and brother…"

This excuse is right along the same line as inherited gum disease. Certainly, it's prudent of me to report the role of host resistance. I hesitate to discuss host resistance to dental disease because I believe that most of the population would simply love to blame their problems on their inability to resist dental disease. They'd rather look me in the eye and report: "bad teeth run in my family."

I rarely meet a patient who will readily admit their own neglect. And when I do, it's so much easier to turn the disease process around.

Once again, let's set the facts straight. Teeth are not "soft"; in fact, enamel is the strongest substance in the human body, stronger than bone. If you've had problems with your teeth ever since you were a kid, perhaps you should decrease your sugar intake, temper your intake of acidic foods (soda and coffee will dissolve enamel and make you more susceptible to tooth decay) and undoubtedly you should spend more time with your toothbrush, dental floss, and your dentist!

"I have TMJ…"

This one drives me nuts! Again, this boils down to education. Educated patients appreciate their dentist more, return and refer more! I'm uncertain how gross anatomy is being taught today, but in defense of the older dentists, we didn't dissect the temporo-mandibular joint in that class.

Whose brainy idea was that? I had to study this extremely important joint – the most complicated in the human body due to its ability to move in different directions so we can chew, and speak – on my own, post-graduation. I worked hard to understand its function and find knowledgeable clinicians to coach me and answer my questions.

So, let's talk about what "TMJ" really is. First, please abandon the term "TMJ" - that's simply the name of the joint and all mammals have two of them: one on the right, the other on the left. When you have issues with your TMJ, you have TMD: Temporo-mandibular *Dysfunction*. Whether from clenching, grinding or an accident, without treatment you will undoubtedly pass through several stages until you are bone-on-bone. Again, I know this from personal experience.

I've completely destroyed my temporo-mandibular joints. As a kid living in an extremely stressful environment, I clenched and bruxed (another term for grinding) my teeth so hard that upon waking I could literally hear the contracted muscle fibers around my ears as they worked to relax. It was a humming sound, and at the time, I didn't understand what was happening, which prompted me to learn more as I passed from one stage of joint dysfunction to where I am today: bone-on-bone.

"I Use an Electric Toothbrush!"

When patients say this to me as if it's some sort of badge of excellence, I'm always so tempted to say, "So?" Why do you patients who buy an "electric toothbrush" think this precludes you from dental disease? I wish I had a dollar for every time I had to say, "A toothbrush is only as good as the person holding it." It's not a get-out-of-jail-free card or some magical ingredient that promises a great dental check-up.

If you use it correctly, great. But if you brush fast and furious with it, it doesn't matter. If you only brush in the morning and do it fast and furious, a dozen electric toothbrushes won't improve your dental health. Again, use it correctly and it can make a difference, but a good manual toothbrush can do the same thing, it just takes longer. My opinion only, but I've peered into thousands of mouths to arrive at it.

"I'm changing dentists because my dentist did substandard care."

I recently had a conversation with a friend who was working with me on my home renovation. He said he was changing dentists because he felt his dentist was doing "substandard work." I asked him how he knew that, and he said he had a post and crown placed and it "came out in two years." I asked him if the doctor had initially suggested an implant and a crown, to which he stated, "Yes, it had been an option," adding, "The cost was about four thousand dollars!"

I also asked if the doctor had told him there was no guarantee of the longevity of the post/crown option, and the answer to that was yes as well. I asked him if the dentist had suggested the implant was a better long-term option – another yes.

Tell me: how do you determine a doctor of dentistry does substandard work if he or she gave you two options, no guarantee of longevity of the cheaper of the two options, and the cheaper option failed in two years? The guy hadn't been to the dentist in those two years and if I were to guess, he didn't floss either – yet somehow it's all the doctor's fault? Wow! Again, we cannot win. Whenever I hear of people foregoing the recommended treatment because of cost, I hear my mother's words: "Always, always, always buy quality. You will spend less in the end."

I lost all the calcium in my teeth when I got pregnant with my kids...

Sorry, not a chance. Calcium ions come in and out of your long bones. Once teeth are formed, the only thing removing calcium is acid erosion (created by you) and acid from aerobic bacterial activity causing tooth decay (also created by you). Never does anyone lose the calcium just because they get pregnant. Come on, God is way smarter than that.

CHAPTER TWENTY-ONE

OBSTACLES TO EXCELLENT CARE

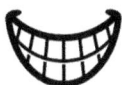

Have you ever thought about what might impede a dentist, hygienist, or assistant from doing an excellent job? There are so many things that can happen and I'm certain you've never even given it a thought. The first thing that comes to mind is the giant mustache that folds down over the upper lip and covers all the upper front teeth and half the opening of your mouth.

I have told patients I need them to trim their mustaches in order to do their dentistry. Some comply, while others refuse; still others just forget to do it prior to their appointment (which has sharpened my trimming skills significantly!). Whatever the case, if I can't see what I am doing, it's not happening. Our work is hard enough without the added encumbrance of their facial hair.

Turn off your cell phone and put it away from your eyes and hands. Why do you think I can work while you text or watch a movie? Really? You lift your phone up between the light and your mouth and you think that's okay? To say nothing about all your movement while my handpiece moves at 30,000 RPMs!

Oh, and don't giggle your feet either. Have you ever dropped a pebble in a still pool of water? The motion ripples out over a large area. When you jiggle your feet, your head moves even more! It's tough to hit a moving target. So please, sit still! The more you cooperate, the faster you'll get out of here.

"I can't open any farther!" In some cases, this is true; this may require a consultation with an oral surgeon regarding a problem with your jaw joint. Truth be told, some divas (and I mean women) just won't cooperate, and I clearly saw you laughing in the reception area with your mouth wide open! It's okay, though. I will do only what you will allow me to, and nothing more.

And let me say this: dentistry is labor-intensive. After fifty-plus years bending over patients and placing myself in any position necessary to get the job done, I hurt. My neck hurts, my back hurts and my hands aren't as pliable as they used to be. After being one of two doctors doing surgery my last few years in dentistry, my right thumb is painfully compromised. There are few retired dentists who might not have remembered the physical nature of dentistry if their neck, back, shoulders and hands didn't continually remind them.

And why do some women come into their early morning dental appointment with lipstick on? I will either smear it all over your face or you'll have to take it off. Think about it! Don't put it on until after the appointment!

I'm not trying to beat a dead horse, but we can't focus on the task at hand if you bring your kids and think you can rock their stroller, continuously give them direction, hold them on your lap, or anything else you're expecting to do while you get your dental treatment done.

Timeliness. Patients get to their dental appointment late, then they want to go to the bathroom and spend several minutes in there brushing their teeth. First, don't brush right before your appointment, it creates a strong saliva flow, making our job more difficult. Second, would you like me to rush through your treatment so I can remain on time for my next patient? Or would you prefer to make the next patient wait while I complete your work?

Most dental offices run behind schedule for one of two reasons: because a patient came late and put them behind, or there was an emergency. When patients arrive at their appointment late, they may as well just say they have no respect for the work we do. Furthermore, a dear friend of mine told me that rushing to any appointment shows disrespect for yourself. Do everyone, including yourself, a favor and plan to show up on time, ready to get down to business.

I've had the pleasure of sitting in a dental chair and receiving treatment on numerous occasions throughout my long life. I've had orthodontic treatment (braces) twice, root canal treatments, extractions (you know, the 'wisdom teeth' we get when we have zero wisdom), and a plethora of fillings on teeth now restored with crowns.

As I sat at my last appointment, I was reminded how uncomfortable receiving dental treatment can be. *However*, I also realized my dentist can't do his part if I don't do mine. I strongly recommend clinicians document these types of obstacles clearly and consistently. When treatment doesn't go as planned because the patient's behavior or attitude is an obstacle, your best defense, should a defense be needed, is your documentation.

CHAPTER TWENTY-TWO

OTHER ISSUES, DESPITE EXCELLENT HOME CARE

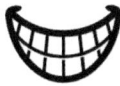

The patients who walk in and readily admit they created their own dental problems are patients I'm most eager to help. They listen, they heed my words, and they work to change their behavior and attitude about their oral health. Indeed, these are rare people.

Then there are the patients to whom, despite good-to-great home care, stuff still happens. Accidents that chip or injure the health of the front teeth are somewhat common. Over the years they've had several treatments to "fix" the tooth that has fractured, or one that has gotten darker because of pulpal death. External whitening doesn't work, it just makes the tooth look darker because the teeth around them get bleached and appear whiter.

Internal bleaching helps a great deal if the injury is fresh, but first, you'll need a root canal treatment to block the bleach from getting to the bone at and out the end of the tooth. The tooth can be bleached from the inside, bringing the natural color back to close to where it was prior to the injury and if you're super lucky, *remarkably close* to the original color.

If you chip a front tooth, you'll likely be diagnosed for either a crown or a filling. Don't choose a filling if your function, habits, and home care are working against it. And for heaven's sake, don't do a filling just because it's cheaper! It discolors over time, it wears, and there's probably no guarantee it will stay in place long term.

Vertical fractures are a huge problem! If your tooth sustains a fracture that runs down under bone, the tooth is history. Period. There's no fixing a vertical fracture and the only solution is to 1) leave the space (which as I've already said carries with it problems in the future); 2) place a bridge, which means cutting down the teeth on either side of the space (Remember once a tooth is prepped it's irreversible); or 3 place an implant. An implant may mean lifting your sinus cavity and implants take time to fuse with bone. Decisions, decisions!

Then there's the oh, so prevalent problem of acid erosion. Really, I'd call it an epidemic as there's hardly a patient I saw towards the end of my career who didn't have some degree of acid erosion. Never heard of it? Here's how it works...

Carbonated beverages are acidic, even if they are sugar-free. Add the problem of sugar and you have a real war going on in your mouth. Coffee, coffee, tea! These habit-forming beverages are highly acidic, and they are dissolving the enamel of your teeth when consumed in heavy doses. Let's add grinding your teeth, and for some of you that's day and night. Now you've softened the enamel and you're going to stress it even more! Not only does that wear your teeth, now you're also taxing your jaw joint.

Other acidic consumptions include fruit. One of the biggest issues I saw was patients placing fresh lemon juice into their drinking water. I did some quick research and found the following list of fruits and their pH from <u>Clemson University</u>[5]. Here they are, from the most acidic to least:

lemon juice (pH: 2.00–2.60)
limes (pH: 2.00–2.80)
blue plums (pH: 2.80–3.40)
grapes (pH: 2.90–3.82)
pomegranates (pH: 2.93–3.20)
grapefruits (pH: 3.00–3.75)
blueberries (pH: 3.12–3.33)
pineapples (pH: 3.20–4.00)
apples (pH: 3.30–4.00)
peaches (pH: 3.30–4.05)
oranges (pH: 3.69–4.34)
tomatoes (pH: 4.30–4.90)

If a neutral pH is 7, and 2 is highly acidic, then eating healthy can be overly acidic. For the health of your teeth, rinse, rinse, and rinse some more after eating. It will dilute the acid. DON'T BRUSH after a meal with a lot of acidic foods. If you brush, you're abrading enamel that has been weakened by the acidic foods…rinse!

_____

[5] https://www.clemson.edu/extension/food/food2market/documents/ph_of_common_foods.pdf

CHAPTER TWENTY-THREE

SHITTY BOSSES

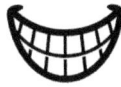

As mentioned earlier, some dentists join existing practices as associate dentists, rather than starting their own practice right out of dental school. Many older dentists find associate dentists who can eventually buy their practice as they approach retirement. For some, this works out well, and for others, not so much. It depends on the intentions of the practice owner in bringing on their younger colleagues.

I was told of a situation where the dentist hired associates so he could just sit in his office, spew orders, and collect the money from his associates' work, giving them a small percentage. The entire plan failed. All his associates quit! In another, the associate dentist was brought on with the intention of selling the practice to them at a given time.

Corporate dentistry can be disappointing. Yes, they offer good benefits, and they manage everything but the dentistry, but oftentimes they don't care about the dentist (or the patient); they just push production, production, production. Make no mistake: they are in the business of making money; dentistry is simply the vehicle. I admit, I'm not very adept at ass-kissing, so this was difficult for me.

Then there's the associate who discovers his boss is sleeping with not one, but two of his employees. In the story I heard, the favoritism displayed caused seven key employees to quit. He cried while begging a couple of them to stay.

How about the receptionist and her best friend, the office manager of a corporate practice, altering a treatment plan procedure? In this situation a large filling had been planned, but the receptionist, after discussing it with the patient, changed the treatment to a crown! She then told the dentist (who is simply an employee but *fully* liable for treatment): "We know what our patients need."

The only problem with that is that the receptionist is not a licensed Doctor of Dentistry. The liability for over-diagnosing falls directly on the dentist, even though he was also an employee. Besides, who does a crown on an eighty-nine-year-old patient with severe heart disease, when a good filling will suffice? Shameful!

I received another story about two female dentists who were accused of discriminating against a new assistant based on her sexual orientation. The two dentists had a *similar* version of events, namely, that the assistant kept interrupting conversations she was having with patients and parents of young patients. This assistant repeatedly gave inappropriate information, performed procedures outside the area her certification allowed, was outwardly defiant of instruction, and displayed an attitude of superiority. The initial dentist asked her colleague if she would mind switching assistants as she thought it was just a personality clash.

Unfortunately, the situation remained the same, resulting in the refusal of both dentists to work with the assistant. When the assistant reported their "bias," it became clear the company was only looking out for the company and wouldn't protect the doctors in any way. Both dentists quit and pursued employment elsewhere.

Patients have no idea this stuff goes on behind the scenes! What an impediment to excellent care!

In another practice, the associate dentist was highly suspicious of the wife of the owner dentist, who was altering completed treatment to reflect services that demanded a higher fee when processed through the insurance company. In plain language, this is called insurance fraud. The one caveat is that the associate dentist can be considered liable as well, even as an employee. I recommended that he leave the practice immediately.

I've worked for two specialists in my career, and the last one belongs in this chapter. Whenever I have been hired as an associate, across the board, I'm asked to let the manager know if there is anything I need to complete the work I was hired to do. You can put five dentists in a room and ask them how they do a composite filling, and no two answers will be the same. The procedure may be similar, but the brands of materials used, and the instruments needed to accomplish the procedure will vary to some degree.

In this practice, I clearly reported I was not the specialist, had done some of this specialized dentistry and was very willing to add to my limited knowledge. The problem was, I was not allowed to use my own methods, but was required to do the procedures exactly as he did them. Long story short, there were procedures I did he did not like, and it simply didn't work out. However, instead of coaching and mentoring me, he shamed me.

So different was he from Dr. Gaspard, DDS, who as mentioned earlier, my mentor as a young dentist. When I first opened my practice and I wasn't busy, I worked part-time for him. I still recall the day he came up to my left shoulder, put his arms around me (something we would never do today!), and said: "You're so damn good, I'm going to push you as far as you will allow me to." Rest in peace, Dr. G, you were amongst the absolute best, and I was blessed to have had you in my corner!

EPILOGUE

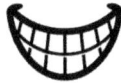

In closing, find a dentist you trust and treat them well. They, in turn, will treat you with the best skills they have developed. Unless they ask otherwise, call them by their much-earned name as Dr. So-and-So. Show up on time, cooperate, heed their recommendations, and pay your bill on your way out the door.

Hopefully, you're better informed of what he or she has gone through after reading this little book. Did you recognize yourself anywhere on these pages? Maybe I made you laugh out loud and maybe not. I was just trying to get you to see things from our side for a change!

In the best dental practices, the dental team is highly valued by the practice owner. Please don't whine when the dental assistant puts on a smile and ushers you back for your appointment. They don't need to hear how much you hate being there and remember: you might be one of those patients they don't care for either. As auxiliaries, they may not have sacrificed as much to gain their title, but they work hard for you and for the practice.

A big thank you to my patients who appreciated me, and my effort to always do my best. I know I could have been a little OCD, but in dentistry, I happen to think that's a good thing!

Yours For Better Health,

Dr. Marynak

ACKNOWLEDGMENTS

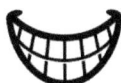

Mr. Thomas A. Lundquist

My true love and life partner who has cheered me on after watching me sit for hours pounding these keys on my computer. Thank you, Tommy!

Mr. Marcus Masters

One of my best and dearest friends, an unlikely duo we are! My highly intelligent, and articulate twenty-six- year-old friend was the very first to read this book. His high compliments had me walking three feet off the floor. Thank you, Marcus!

Dr. Juris Purins, MD

I'd like to thank Dr. Juris Purins. I met Dr. Purins at the University of Minnesota School of Dentistry in 1980.

It wasn't long before he quit dental school and decided on medical school because he thought dental school was too difficult. I still recall sitting in his apartment and playing Pac Man (now I'm dating myself!). I was beating him and can still hear him saying that I had excellent eye-hand coordination, whereby I almost said: "dah, I'm a dental student!"

After graduation, we were sitting at a coffee shop in St. Paul, Minnesota, discussing what the name of this book should be. It was Juris who said: "Down in the Mouth Again." I can only own the last half of the title. Thank you, Dr. Purins, MD!

My Dental Friends and Colleagues

My too numerous to name, group of friends and colleagues who have donated their stories. They donated the good, the bad, and the ugly. Thank you to all my friends and colleagues for your input!

ABOUT THE AUTHOR

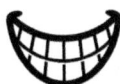

D r. Deborah L. Marynak began her career in dentistry as a dental technician in the field of "porcelain jacket crowns" in 1970. In 1972, she began preparing to become a dental hygienist. and graduated from Normandale Community College, School of Dental Hygiene in 1976. Within the year, she began her pre-dental studies and entered the University of Minnesota, School of Dentistry in 1980.

Since graduating from dental school in 1984, she's owned and operated her private practice for 20 years. She's worked as an associate in both Wisconsin and Oregon. In Wisconsin, she also worked as the supervising dentist for the Ho-Chunk Healthcare Clinic in Black River Falls. She's gained experience in corporate, nursing home, and prison dentistry.

She started a company called DentalStaffing.org in 2015 with a goal of helping Dental Professionals find the right fit for both the employee and the employer. She's also developed a site to help patients understand their recommended dental treatment: DentalHealthToday.com

She has worked with dental offices to help them streamline their clinical systems and has taught dental teams how to effectively document patient charts to avoid risk. She is a strong believer in sound systems, and all systems begin and end with a strong, cohesive Team. Her work has been with dentists, hygienists, assistants, dental office managers, administrative staff, and their dental labs, both individually and with entire Teams.

Dr Marynak is now retired from clinical dentistry, and living in North Carolina. She still owns and operates www.DentalStaffing. org. In her spare time, she likes to spend time with her four-legged kids (four dogs and two cats.) gardening, and antiquing. She loves what most people see as junk; if it's rusty metal or has peeling paint, she probably wants it.